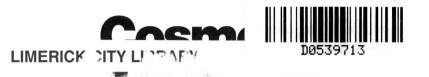
One to one massage

For Mum, Dad, Marcelle and S.J.P - thanks for your encouragement, love and support.

Eve Cameron

To Ma, Pa and Claire for their love; to Mike for his inspiration; and especially to Marty and Shannon Emerald Georgia for seeing me through another one with such patience!

Karena Callen

Thanks also to Stephen Russell and Madeleine Burbidge for their technical help on, respectively, the Sensual Massage and Shiatsu chapters.

Cosmopolitan

One to one massage

expert techniques to relax and stimulate

Eve Cameron & Karena Callen

Massage consultant:
Isabelle Hughes, London College of Massage
Additional research and text:
Saskia Sarginson

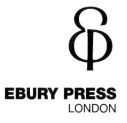

EBURY PRESS
LONDON

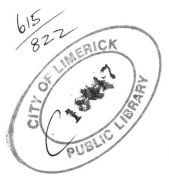

First published 1993
1 3 5 7 9 10 8 6 4 2
Text © National Magazine Company Ltd 1993
Photography © Ebury Press 1993

First published in the United Kingdom in 1993 by
Ebury Press, Random House, 20 Vauxhall Bridge Road,
London SW1V 2SA

Random House Australia (Pty) Limited
20 Alfred Street, Milsons Point, Sydney
New South Wales 2061, Australia

Random House New Zealand Limited
18 Poland Road, Glenfield
Auckland 10, New Zealand

Random House South Africa (Pty) Limited
PO Box 337, Bergvlei, South Africa

Random House UK Limited Reg. No. 954009

A CIP catalogue record for this book is available from the British Library.

Photography Oliver Pearce

Design Shirley Saphir, Jerry Goldie
Editor Joanna Bradshaw
Styling Eve Cameron and Karena Callen
Hair Karin Darnell and Suzanna Perks,
using Paul Mitchell Luxury Haircare
Make-up Karin Darnell and Suzanna Perks
Illustrations Tony Hannaford

ISBN 0 09 177703 8

Typeset by Textype Typesetters, Cambridge,
and by Clive Dorman & Co., London
Printed in Great Britain by Butler & Tanner Ltd, Frome and London

WARNING
If you have a medical condition, or are pregnant, the massages
described in this book should not be followed without first consulting
your doctor. All guidelines and warnings should be read carefully and
the authors and publisher cannot accept responsibility for injuries or
damage arising out of a failure to comply with the same.

contents

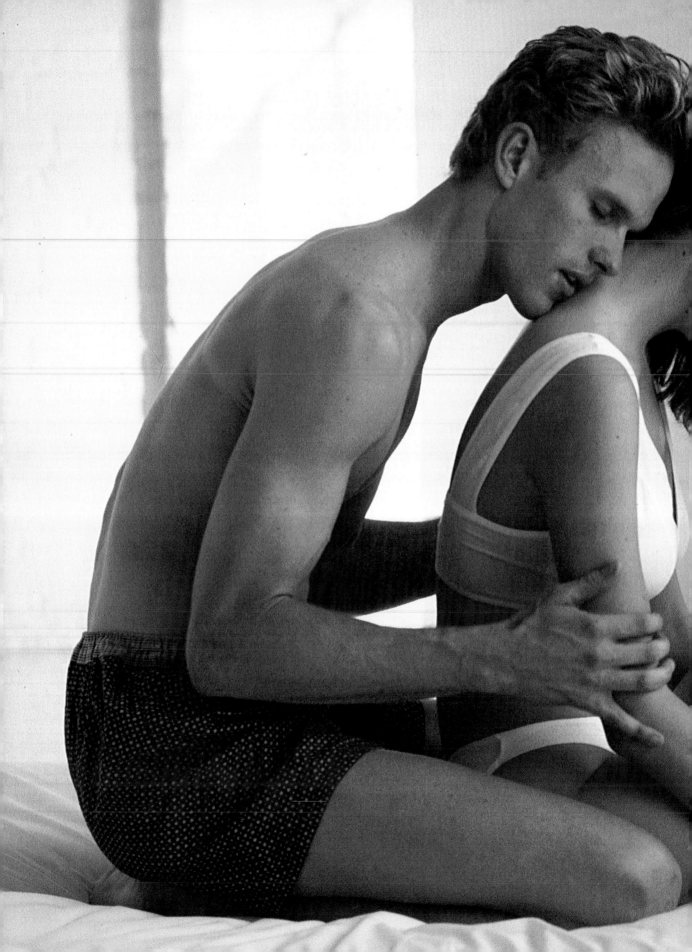

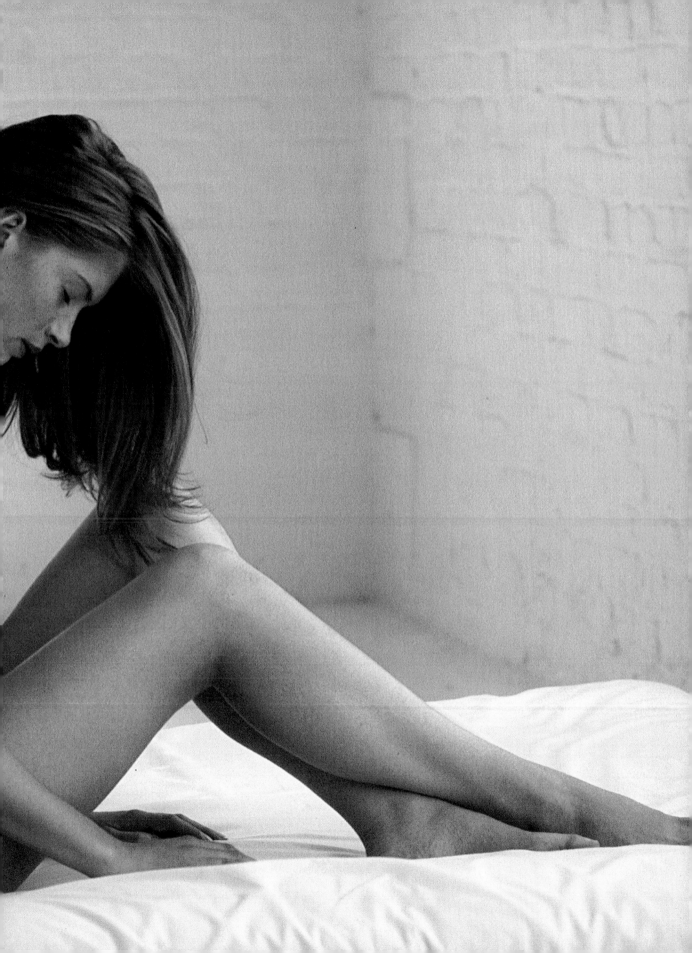

introduction

Touch is vital to both our physical and emotional well being. Apart from our sense of smell, touch is the most important of the senses for establishing strong bonds in our relationships. For example, it's essential for a newborn baby to experience the reassuring touch of its mother in order to grow into a healthy individual. And indeed any close relationship is enhanced and maintained with frequent touching.

Massage is really just an extension of our primitive instinct to touch and be touched. It helps us to relax and unwind and eases aches and pains. The medical profession has now proved that massage has far-reaching physiological effects on the body. For example, it has been shown to trigger the release of endorphins, natural pain-killers produced by the brain, that help to block pain and produce feelings of euphoria and contentment. On another level, massage also helps us tune in to our emotional and spiritual self.

Although massage is really an intuitive art, its practitioners through the centuries have worked hard at perfecting its basic strokes in order to achieve optimum results. The ancient Greeks were especially fond of massage and believed that it had potent healing powers. It was used then as it is now, by athletes and other sportspeople before and after training and competitions, to help heal injuries and to promote relaxation. The Romans also recognized its therapeutic effects. Galen, the famous physician, wrote a series of books detailing the benefits of touch. He even described a variety of strokes, "I direct that the strokes and circuits of the hands should be made of many sorts, in order that as far as possible all muscle fibres should be rubbed in every direction."

However, it was the ancient Chinese and Japanese who developed some of the most popular techniques. Shiatsu, acupressure and reflexology all stem from the East, although they have been adopted and adapted by Western therapists. Even the so-called Swedish massage has been influenced in part by eastern techniques. Per Henrik Ling, a physiologist, developed the basis of this now internationally used method while travelling in China in the late 18th and early 19th centuries. On his return to Sweden he combined these basic strokes with his own movements to create an original and effective method that was more in tune with Western needs.

Swedish massage is used as the basis for the first section of this book. Five of these chapters are divided into areas of the body – head, neck and shoulders; face; back; hands, arms and stomach; and bottom, legs and feet. In each, you'll find stages which, when combined, form a total body massage. Follow them as a sequence through the chapters or use them individually to concentrate on one area. There are also do-it-yourself techniques throughout, as well as quick pick-me-ups that take only a few minutes to perform. We've also included a chapter on aromatherapy. This features a separate face and body routine, but you could also use the aromatherapy tips in combination with the basic Swedish moves.

In the second section of the book, we explore some other forms of massage. These are sensual sequences to practise with your partner and introductions to reflexology and shiatsu. Each of these is of course worth a book on its own, but we hope you'll learn a lot from these tasters of the techniques.

Enjoy...

Eve Cameron and Karena Callen

part 1

swedish massage aroma

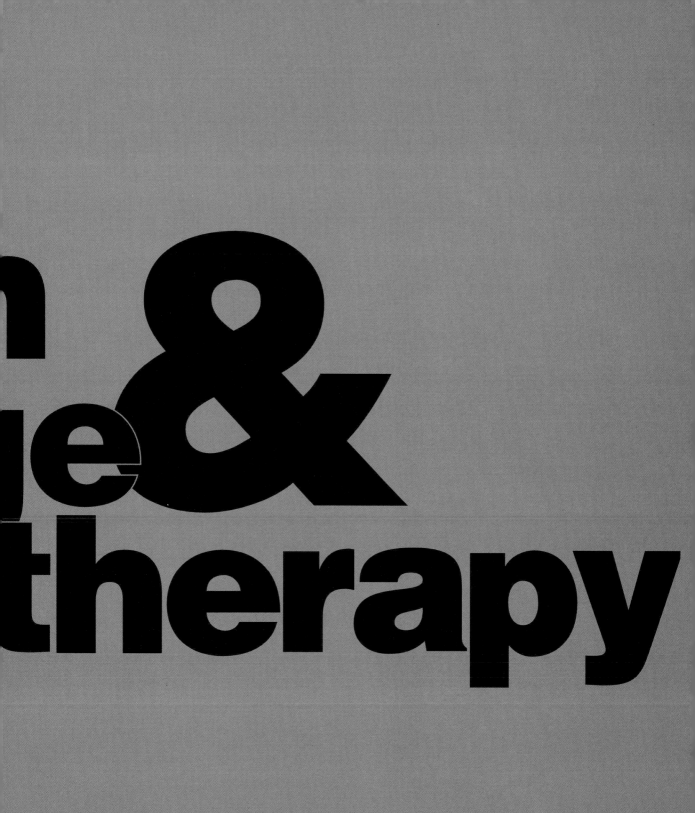

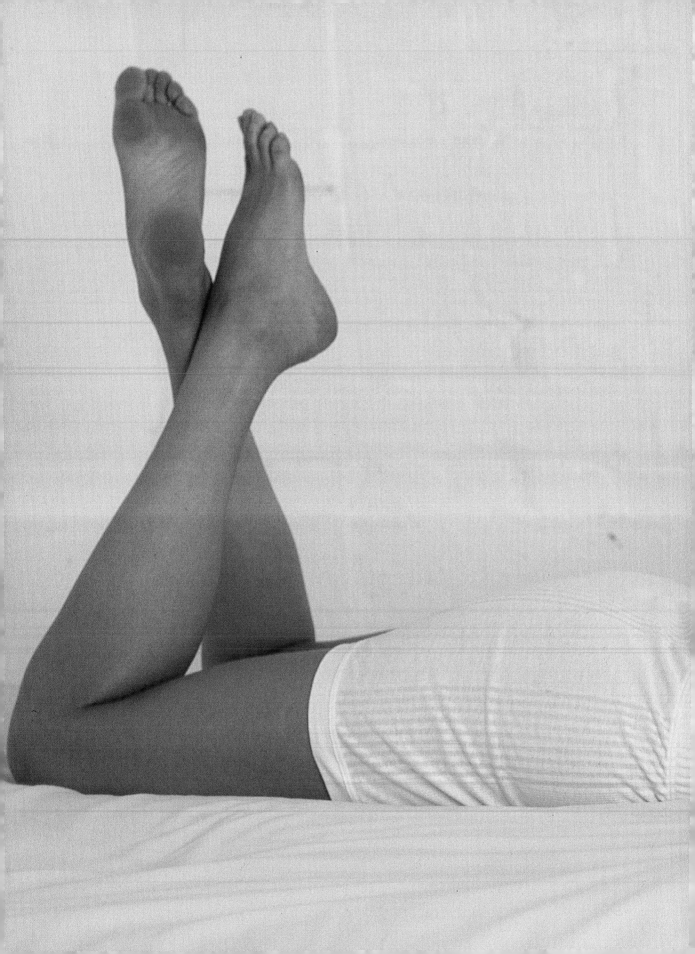

basics

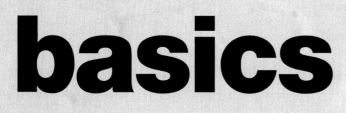

the aim of swedish massage is to maintain or restore good health through specific and careful manipulation of the joints and muscles.

The idea of massage for health was reintroduced to Europe in the late 18th and early 19th centuries by a Swede, Per Henrik Ling, who believed in combining massage with 'medical gymnastics'. His treatments were made up of passive and gymnastic movements – the latter often involving quite a lot of physical activity on the part of the massage giver. As a result of his influential work, a Swedish Institute was opened in London in 1838 and by the end of the century other such institutes had been established all over Europe and in the United States.

The strokes Ling advocated included pressure, friction, vibration, percussion and rotation – the basis, in fact, of the strokes many massage practitioners use today. Thankfully Ling's techniques have been refined somewhat, losing the exercise aspect of the original Swedish massage. It is now an altogether more relaxing process for both parties. But, while the techniques may have changed – there are four main movements used in this type of massage – effleurage, petrissage, friction and tapotement – the massage you're likely to receive in a beauty salon or at a health club may well be referred to as Swedish massage.

In addition to the usual massage practitioners in beauty salons and leisure centres, many doctors and nurses are also trained in massage nowadays. Research has shown it to be beneficial not only to people who are recovering in hospital, but also to those with terminal diseases such as cancer, easing their pain on both a physical and a mental level.

making the most of massage

One of the best things about massage is that you can do it anywhere, for any length of time. From a quick fifteen minute pick-me-up for neck and shoulders in the office or a heavenly foot massage on the beach, to five minutes self-massage on your face or a leisurely full body massage – the potential is endless.

When giving or receiving a total body massage that is supposed to be soothing and relaxing (though you can make it stimulating too by using certain essential oils and specific massage moves), your environment is most important. In fact, your surroundings could make the difference between an agreeable rub and a truly restorative experience.

creating the mood

It is essential that you create a peaceful, calming atmosphere before embarking on a full massage sequence. Don't allow yourself to be disturbed or distracted in any way. It's worthwhile unplugging the telephone and maybe even locking the door before you start. Music can be useful in helping you to relax. Classical and New Age music in particular are wonderfully soothing if you both like them. Silence can be just fine too.

Make sure the room is warm – it's hard to relax in a cold or draughty environment. Even though the person receiving the massage is usually covered up, with the exception of the part of their body on which you are working, it's a good idea to have extra blankets and towels on hand for added warmth. A heater may be useful too as massage causes the body temperature to drop slightly as your partner relaxes. After working on one area of the body, the muscles there should be kept warm and covered up with a towel or blanket. (*Note*: In the photographs the person receiving the massage is uncovered so that the moves can be seen clearly.)

Lighting is important too; it should not be too harsh as it's hard to relax under bright lights. Candlelight is perfect (especially for sensual massage, see pages 92–101), while strong sunlight should be filtered and electric light is best dimmed.

the massage surface

The ideal place for a full massage is the floor, softened a bit and made comfortable with a folded duvet, several layers of blankets or towels, or a slimline hard mattress or futon. If you're massaging someone on the floor, remember to place a cushion or some folded towels under your knees, otherwise they will really suffer. A solid table at a workable height is another possibility, again made more comfortable with a layer of blankets. If you are massaging on a regular basis, a lightweight portable couch is a useful investment.

Many people believe that the most obvious place to use as a massage surface is a bed. It is in fact the

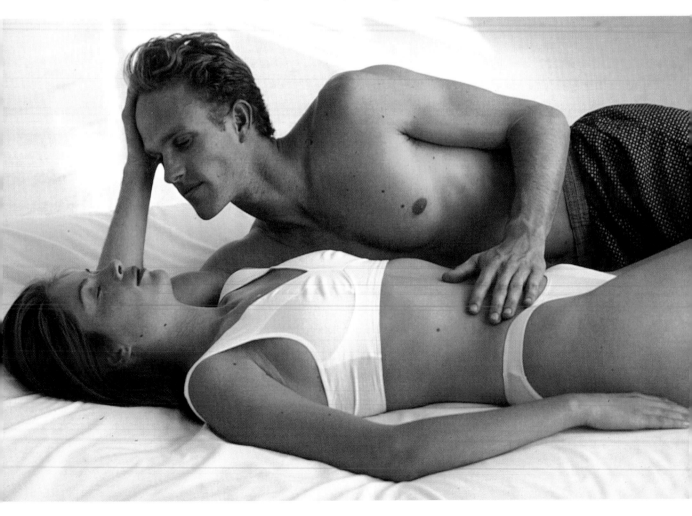

worst possible choice, for two reasons: firstly, mattresses are usually too soft and will give as you apply pressured movements, making them less effective. Secondly, beds are invariably at just the wrong height and are likely to give backache to whoever is doing the massage.

massage preparation

● **massage giver** Wear comfortable clothes and remove any jewellery that could be noisy and distracting or scratch the person you're massaging. If you have mid-length or long hair, tie it back. Check the length of your nails too – talons are impossible to work with. It is essential that you are completely relaxed before you give a massage, as you have to offer your full attention, care and concentration. If you are tense you will find it difficult to massage and it will not feel as relaxing as it could for the recipient either. To prepare yourself mentally, just sit and relax for a few minutes. Breathe deeply and clear your mind before starting work.

● **massage recipient** It is easier to massage a naked body rather than to have to work around straps and seams. However it is important that you feel secure whilst being massaged, so whatever level of undress feels right for you is the most appropriate. If you're being massaged by a close friend or partner, nudity probably won't be an issue. Remove all jewellery for comfort and safety and so as not to impede the flow of the massage. Help yourself relax by breathing deeply, then tensing and consciously untensing all your muscles. Alternatively, take a deep breath and, as you exhale, let your body sink into the floor and become as limp as possible.

where to start?

It's up to you (and your partner) which area of the body you start on when performing a total body massage. Obviously you should avoid turning someone from their back to their stomach and vice versa more than once during a session. A suggested sequence is to start with the receiver on his or her back, work on the buttocks and the backs of the legs, ask the person to turn, then work on the feet, then the front of the legs and progress up the body to finish on the face. Alternatively, you could massage in exactly the reverse direction. Wherever you start, try to ensure that the movements flow together and that you completely finish one area before moving on to the next. Remember to keep the body covered all the time, except for the area you're massaging, unless conditions are ideal and it is warm enough to leave the body uncovered.

For continuity of flow and to keep the massage recipient feeling secure, always keep one hand in contact with their body – even if you have to stop for more oil or to change your own position. And, another tip, never pour oil straight out of its container onto someone's skin – they'll get a cold shock. It should be poured out into your hand first so that your body heat warms it.

The basic strokes of massage and numerous step-by-step techniques are described in the following chapters, but remember to trust your intuition too – your hands are natural, powerful healing tools.

contraindications

Massage is an enjoyable and valuable therapy, but there are certain contraindications that you should be aware of.

● **pregnancy**

Whilst massage is a fabulous relaxation aid and ache-soother for the mother-to-be (many experts say it positively influences the well-being of the baby too), care must be taken with her abdomen and lower back. Never use strong pressure on either – percussion movements are best avoided too. If using essential oils, remember that some are contraindicated during pregnancy because of the risk of miscarriage (see page 82). Safe choices for pregnant women include lavender and tangerine.

● **varicose veins**

Use light stroking movements only, or, if the condition is very severe and you are in doubt, avoid the area completely. If clots are found in the veins, strong massage could cause them to move, with potentially fatal consequences.

● **high fever**

A massage will not calm a fever. Rest, plenty of fluids and medical advice are recommended instead.

● **infectious skin disorders**

Scabies, ringworm and athlete's foot are examples of infectious skin conditions which could be spread or transferred to you as a result of massage.

● **recent surgery/scars**

Massage, unless performed by a professional, could lead to complications so is best avoided. Old scars can safely be massaged over. Likewise, minor wounds, such as bites or scratches, are not a problem.

carrier oils

Oil greatly helps the smooth and flowing movements of massage. Of course, if you're giving someone a quick neck rub at the office while they have turned off their computer for ten minutes, oil will be far too messy; besides, one layer of clothing will give a little bit of 'slip'. In most situations though, your massage technique will be made easier with the use of oil, and you won't drag the skin of the person you're massaging. Oil will also condition the skin.

To apply oil to your hands, pour about a teaspoon of oil into one palm and then rub your palms together. Repeat before you start to work on each new part of the body.

There are plenty of commercially made massage oils available in shops. Buy these if you find them convenient and like them; you might need to try a few until you find a blend you really like. Equally there are many ways of creating your own blends of oil.

Vegetable oil is a good choice as a carrier, or base, oil. Baby oil (a mineral oil that is a by-product of the petrochemical industry) doesn't absorb

ten massage tips

1. Have you checked for contraindications?
2. Make sure the room is warm and lighting subtle.
3. No disruptions. Chose soothing music or opt for silence – you need to concentrate. Take your cue from the person you're massaging and talk if they want to.
4. Are extra blankets, towels and cushions to hand?
5. Are you both relaxed?
6. Have you removed your jewellery?
7. Have you worked out where to start your sequence?
8. Remember that one of the most important elements of massage is the flow of movement. It should feel rather like following the rhythm of a relaxing piece of music. Just let yourself go.
9. Use pressure differently according to which part of the body you're working on. For example, go more gently on delicate places such as the pelvic area and work more deeply on the thighs and back. Do ask if the pressure you are using feels comfortable.
10. A total body massage should last about an hour and a half. Check first if the person you are massaging would like you to concentrate on any specific areas.

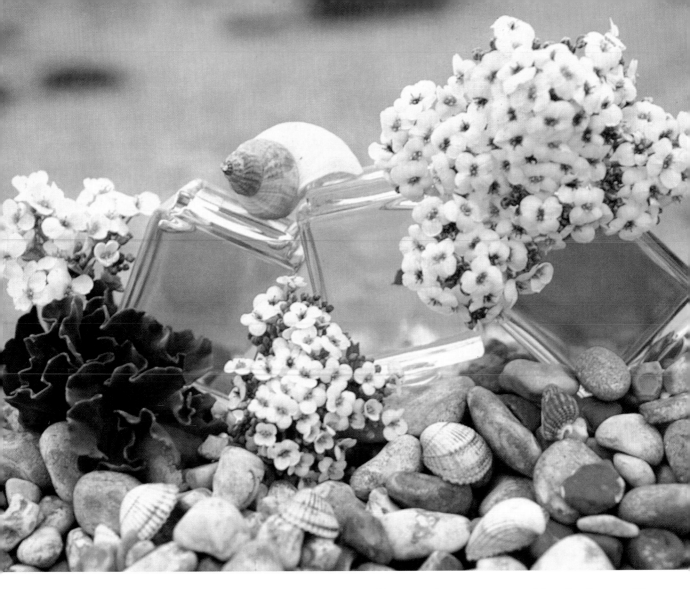

well, so it is not a good medium for essential oils. Your regular body moisturizer, unless it is an oil, will probably absorb too quickly for you to work with and olive oil, while it is good for your heart, does not smell so good on your skin. It is also rather too thick to be a massage oil on its own.

Do remember that oils go rancid in time (you will know they have turned by their smell), so don't mix up litres of a massage blend that will then sit around for months. Instead, make up smaller quantities that will be used up quickly. As an extra precaution, include some wheatgerm oil in the blend as it is an efficient natural preservative.

Once you have made up your oil, store it in a dark coloured glass bottle and keep it in a cool, dark place to prolong its life.

which oil to choose?

All the oils listed below may be used alone or in combination. You can add essential oils to them in a ratio of one drop essential oil to 2 ml (½ tsp) carrier oil, to create an aromatherapy massage (see page 80 for more information on aromatherapy). Essential oils are highly concentrated and, with the exception of tea tree and lavender, should never be used undiluted. They 'dissolve' in oil, hence the term 'carrier oil'. The carrier oil literally takes the essential oils on to the skin and helps them disperse.

● **sweet almond** From the pink-blossomed sweet almond tree. Used for centuries in skincare, it is one of the most popular oils for massage, both facial and body. It has a high vitamin D content.

● **jojoba** Comes from the beans of the jojoba plant and is a relatively new ingredient in skincare. It is anti-bacterial and has a longer shelf-life than many other oils. With a chemical composition close to sebum – the skin's natural lubricating oil – it suits most skin types, but is especially helpful in treating skin problems, from eczema to acne. It's quite expensive, so reserve it for facial massage or to form part of a blend.

● **avocado** Rich and soothing, yet easily absorbed. It's high in vitamins A and D and contains potassium. Good for all but very sensitive skin types, it is especially suitable for mature skin.

● **peach kernel** Nourishing and sweet-smelling, this oil is rich in vitamin E and essential fatty acids. Great for facial massage.

● **grapeseed** Inexpensive and light-textured. Has no odour of its own.

● **sunflower** An excellent base oil for all skin types, it's affordable and easy to find. (Check that it is pure and additive free.)

● **safflower** As above.

● **wheatgerm** Rich in vitamin E, this oil is a natural preservative and anti-oxidant. It helps maintain the elasticity of the skin and is particularly recommended for dry, dehydrated and older skin types. It is used as an additive, not on its own.

warning
If you are following a course of homeopathic treatment, do not use essential oils as well; aromatherapy can counteract the benefits of any homeopathic remedies.

gadgets

When practising on yourself or even on a partner, massage gadgets can be useful aids to relaxation. One of the most important benefits is that they enable you to reach areas of the body that are normally inaccessible when you're performing a DIY massage. Such gadgets are also designed to give optimum results with minimum effort and, because of their shape and weight, help you to maintain a firm, even pressure. What's more, they are less tiring to use than your hands alone, so you can give yourself or your partner a more intensive massage. We've selected a few of the most widely available gadgets.

● **1 back massager** This is excellent to use on yourself for a DIY treat. Tiny wooden balls massage your back, bottom and thighs, helping to boost circulation and to relax tense muscles.

● **2 sisal massager** This massager is great to use as a quick pick-me-up in the shower or bath. Use it in circular movements to massage damp skin. Work upwards from the feet and sweep up the legs, across the buttocks and along the arms, towards the shoulders and across the chest. It's very stimulating and in addition leaves skin soft and smooth. Great at the end of the day when your energy levels have slumped.

● **3 twin ball massage roller** Also known as a Neural Easer, this massage roller is very effective when used on the neck and back. Because of its long handle, it's easy to reach your own neck and back too. Roll it up and down the spine for best results.

● **4 slim foot roller** Use this gadget to stimulate reflex points on your feet easily and effectively. All you do is remove your shoes and socks, place your foot on the roller and move your sole backwards and forwards over it. Because it's very portable, it's ideal to use when travelling, especially on long plane journeys.

● **5 chunky foot roller** Similar to the slim foot roller in principle, it has three rows of wooden beads which help to stimulate reflex points on the soles of the feet. Press your foot onto the roller for deeper pressure.

● **6 anti-stress roller** Similar to the back massager, this roller is used to massage neck, shoulders, back, bottom and thighs. Use brisk rolling to stimulate and slow, gentle rolling to soothe and relax. Ideal for DIY massage at the end of a stressful day or for a quick pick-me-up first thing in the morning.

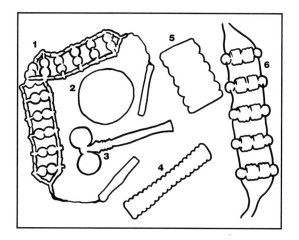

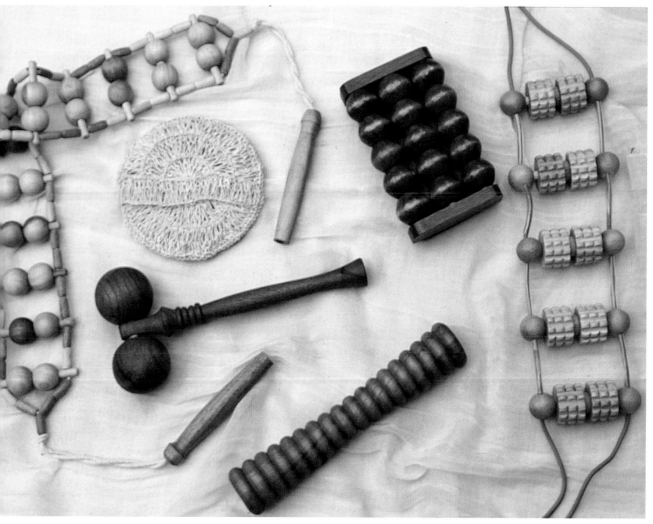

basic strokes

A good massage will unknot muscles, relieve tension and improve circulation and lymphatic drainage. It will bring an instant glow to the skin of the recipient and can either invigorate or relax, depending on the type of strokes applied.

Before you can perform a massage on yourself or a partner, you need to know how to perform the basic strokes.

There are four basic strokes in massage which are as important to a masseur as the five ballet positions are to a dancer – they provide the structure on which the entire art form is based. Learning to use these four basic strokes is the key which will enable you to create a harmonious and complete massage – a massage which will help to soothe, energize and balance your partner's body and mind.

You will find that as your knowledge of the strokes improves, your confidence will grow, and eventually your own intuitive responses will allow you to add a personal touch to these basic massage techniques. One final point to remember, always massage towards the heart – this way, you work with the body's circulatory system.

effleurage

● **the stroke** *Effleurer* means to touch lightly. These are long, gliding strokes which are used to soothe and relax the body. They are generally applied at the start of a massage to gently warm and energize the body, preparing your partner's muscles for deeper, more intensive work later on. Effleurage is also used at the end of a massage to bring the session to a calm, relaxed conclusion.

● **the effect** The gentle, rhythmic stroking of effleurage can act as a sedative on a hyperactive, nervous or anxious partner, and can also help reduce high blood pressure (although this will only be a temporary effect). Featherlight effleurage strokes applied over the forehead, temples and neck have a soothing effect on headaches, migraines or hangovers. If performed over the neck and back – which feels particularly wonderful –

effleurage strokes can help to beat insomnia, sending your partner into a relaxed sleep. However, when effleurage is applied firmly and briskly it will have a stimulating effect, improving blood circulation and helping to detoxify the system. These kind of firm effleurage movements used over muscular injuries will stimulate the lymph flow, helping to reduce any swelling around the injury – but check with a doctor first before massaging recent injuries. Revive tired muscles and give yourself an after-exercise treat with brisk effleurage applied with a refreshing body oil.

● **contraindications** Beware of using effleurage strokes on a partner with a lot of body hair, as the movement could drag at the hair follicles, causing discomfort and a rash. In this

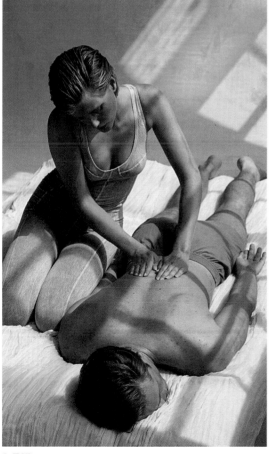

● **Effleurage**

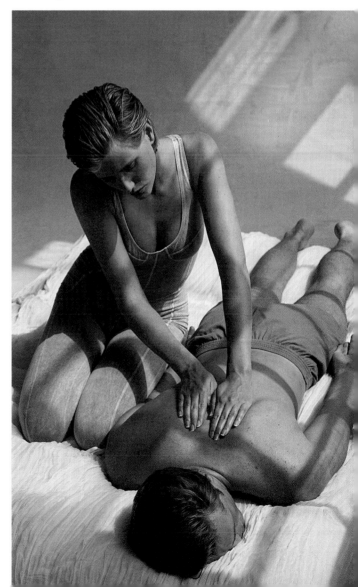

situation, be very generous with the oil. And only apply these strokes very lightly over varicose veins or on sore, inflamed skin.

● **technique** Use the whole of your hands flat on the body, distributing pressure evenly through fingers and palms. Your hands should mould themselves to the shape of your partner's body. Apply the pressure on the upward stroke, creating an even, unbroken sweep across the skin. Lean your body into the stroke from your pelvis, setting up a rhythm within the stroke. When you come to the limit of your natural reach, separate your hands and allow them to trail gently back to your starting point. Let your hands get to know your partner's body through this introductory stroke. Eventually you will learn how to discern areas of tension which you can return to later on in the massage, for more intensive work using another stroke. Contact is never broken between your hands and your partner's body, and when the effleurage movements are over, it is easy to glide into the next technique. You can use effleurage strokes very lightly or with firm pressure, but remember that the character of the stroke should always be smooth and flowing.

petrissage

● **the stroke** An invigorating, refreshing movement that works more deeply on the tissues and more directly with the muscle masses than effleurage. Petrissage derives from the word *petrir*, meaning to knead, and can be applied using several different techniques.

● **the effect** Petrissage increases circulation, warms the area on which you are working, helps cleanse the tissues of accumulated toxins, improves muscle tone and helps break down fatty deposits. It is very effective on fleshy areas such as buttocks and thighs, where it can, if used regularly, help to prevent or reduce cellulite. It can also be used on an area which has recently recovered from a joint or muscle sprain, as it will help to speed the healing process and strengthen the area by increasing blood flow and cleansing the muscles of accumulated metabolic wastes, thus preventing stiffness in the muscles.

● **contraindications** Do not apply

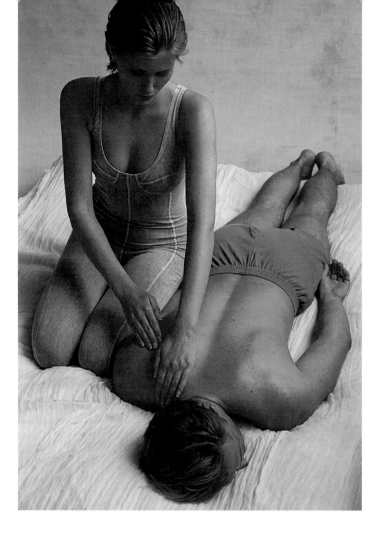

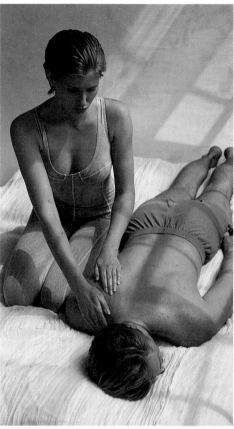

● **Petrissage: wringing**

petrissage strokes over a newly injured area, recent scar tissue, sore or inflamed skin or varicose veins. Also, it is not advisable to use it over the abdomen of someone suffering from gastritis, colitis or any inflammatory condition, or on a pregnant or menstruating woman. Petrissage can otherwise be used everywhere on a healthy body, except the face.

● **techniques** Different petrissage techniques are used according to which part of the body you are work-

ing on. There are three basic techniques as follows:

squeezing This is performed on areas such as the upper shoulder and can be done with one or two hands. Place the fingers under the front of the shoulder and the thumb on top. Pick up and squeeze along the muscles between the shoulder joint and the neck. If you are working on a large area, use both hands alternately.

wringing This is performed on large muscle groups such as the thighs.

Place one hand on the inner thigh and the other on the outer thigh. Push and lift the muscles on both sides in one smooth movement, moving one hand forwards and one hand backwards until your hands have swapped places. Repeat this movement from just above the knee to the top of the thigh. The action can be slow and gentle or firm and vigorous, depending on the needs of your partner and the mood of the massage.

kneading Place both hands on the body over a muscle mass such as the shoulders or buttocks, lean your weight onto one hand, using the whole of the hand to grasp and squeeze the muscle. Then sway your body weight onto the other hand as you squeeze with that hand, letting go of the original hand. In this manner squeeze and knead, working in a rhythmical, rocking style, using your hands in a continuous, alternate action – as if you were kneading bread. Don't worry if the skin you are massaging becomes red and flushed, this signals that blood is now flowing into an area previously blocked by tense muscles. The blood will bring oxygen and nutrients to the area and help clear away accumulated toxins.

Although petrissage is a stimulating stroke, it should never be painful for the recipient.

friction

● **the stroke** Friction strokes penetrate the deeper layers of muscle, affecting the tendons and ligaments around the joints. The action itself is a small, short and controlled application of pressure to a particular area. It is usually applied over specific tight spots and muscle knots.

● **the effect** Friction increases blood flow to the area and loosens fibrous matter and knots. The tissue next to the bone is moved during the stroke and this helps to eliminate waste deposits while stimulating the nerve endings. Friction is particularly good used in bony areas such as the base of the skull, alongside the spine, around the shoulder blades and on the hands and feet.

● **contraindications** Do not use friction over very delicate or sensitive skin. It is also best to steer clear of bruises, recent wounds or scar tissue that is less than six months old.

● **technique** Position yourself

directly above the area you are working on. Using the pad of the thumb, apply pressure downwards over the area of the body to be worked, pressing down slowly and evenly. Apply your own body weight to add controlled depth to the pressure. Hold the pressure for a few seconds before making a tiny, circular movement with the pad of the thumb, then reduce the pressure slowly. Friction is a releasing stroke which eases away tightness and tension. It may hurt so pressure is best applied as your partner breathes out and released as they breathe in.

tapotement

● **the stroke** Tapotement is an energizing stroke best used towards the end of the massage session on a well prepared partner. It will wake and stimulate the body, helping to break down fatty deposits and waste products in the tissue, bringing new suppleness to stiff muscles and improving the tone of slack muscles. The word itself means 'soft drumming' and there are several different tapotement techniques, all of which involve pounding the muscles and skin of the body.

● **the effect** Tapotement has a stimulating, vibratory effect on the body, improving the circulation by attracting blood to the area being worked on and stimulating the nervous system by giving it a series of small shocks. It causes muscle tissue

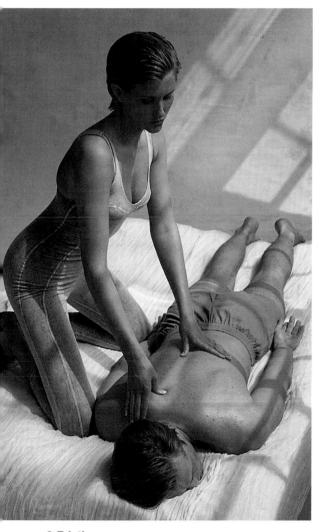

● **Friction**

to contract and draws blood into the skin, helping to tone muscles and refresh the skin. When performed over the back it sets up a vibration which stimulates the skin and internal organs – but do not perform it directly over the spine. On more fleshy parts of the body, like the bottom and the thighs, tapotement can be used on a regular basis to help treat cellulite problems.

● **contraindications** Tapotement is best avoided over bony areas like shins and knees. It should never be used on muscles in spasm, or on very sensitive areas like the calves. Do not

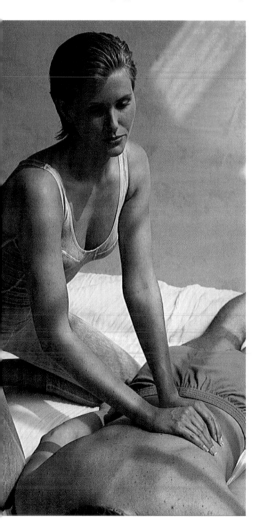

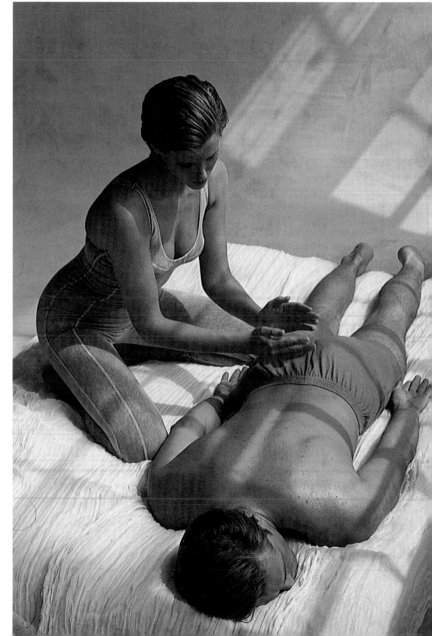

● **Tapotement: cupping** (above), **hacking** (right)

perform tapotement on injured, sore or inflamed skin. If your partner has very sensitive skin all over, you can place a thin towel over the area where you are performing tapotement to help reduce the risk of any possible discomfort.

● techniques

cupping Cup your hands so that the palms and fingers form a hollow curve. Then drum your cupped hands over the skin in a controlled, rhythmical fashion. This should produce a hollow 'clip clop' sound which will tell you that you are performing the stroke correctly – if your hands are too flat they will produce a slapping sound and a stinging effect. Your cupped hands will trap air against the skin, then release it. Use this technique on the back.

pounding Use the underside of your clenched fists to drum over the skin. This stimulates the muscles to contract, thereby tightening and improving muscle and skin tone and really making the skin glow. Maintain a sense of rhythm and keep hands close to the body rather than bouncing them from a height, this will help control both the rhythm and the force that you use. Pounding should be used over fleshy and well muscled areas like the bottom, thighs and calves.

hacking Use the outer edges of your flat hands to flick up and down over the skin in a chopping action, the idea is to perform hacking very rapidly, lightly and rhythmically, moving your hands from the wrists and keeping your arms relaxed.

putting the basic strokes into action

The basic strokes, once learnt and mastered, should always be used in a specific sequence to gain the optimum results from a massage and prevent any chance of discomfort or injury.

1. Effleurage is always used first to relax the muscles and prepare your partner for more intensive work.
2. Petrissage is applied next to begin cleansing the tissues of metabolic wastes.
3. If friction is appropriate to help release specific areas of tension, it should be performed at this point in the massage.
4. Petrissage can be repeated after it.
5. Only now is the body prepared enough for tapotement. Check that your partner hasn't fallen asleep before you begin tapotement, otherwise it will give them a shock.
6. The massage should end with calming effleurage strokes, unless you have applied tapotement, in which case do not use effleurage afterwards. Any break of contact during the massage interrupts the rhythm of the treatment, so make a point of using your hand to maintain contact with your partner's body throughout. This also keeps your partner's sensory nerves stimulated and relaxes the muscle being treated, as well as the person being massaged.

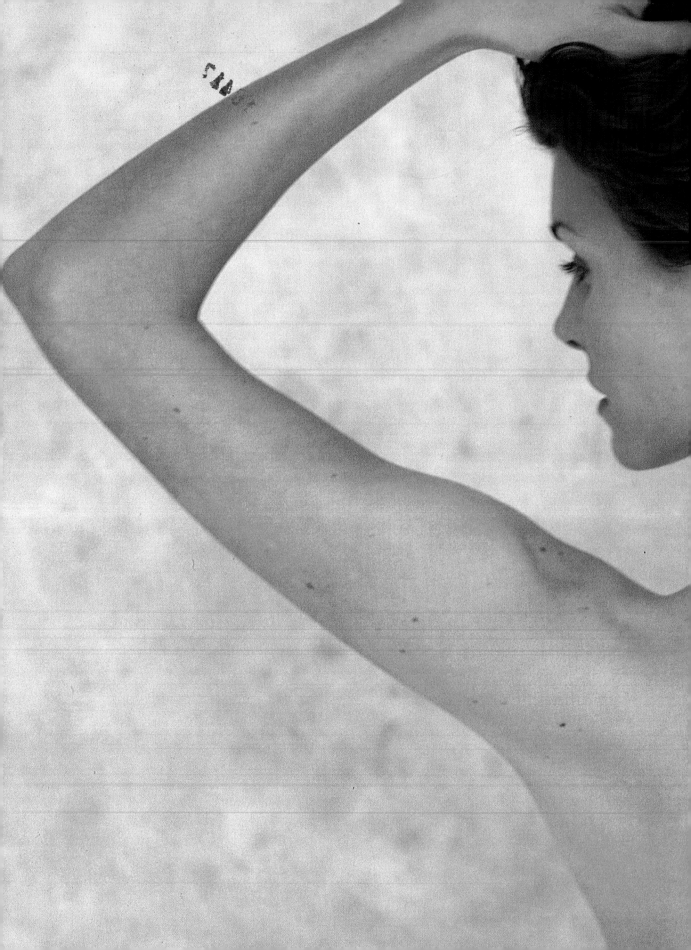

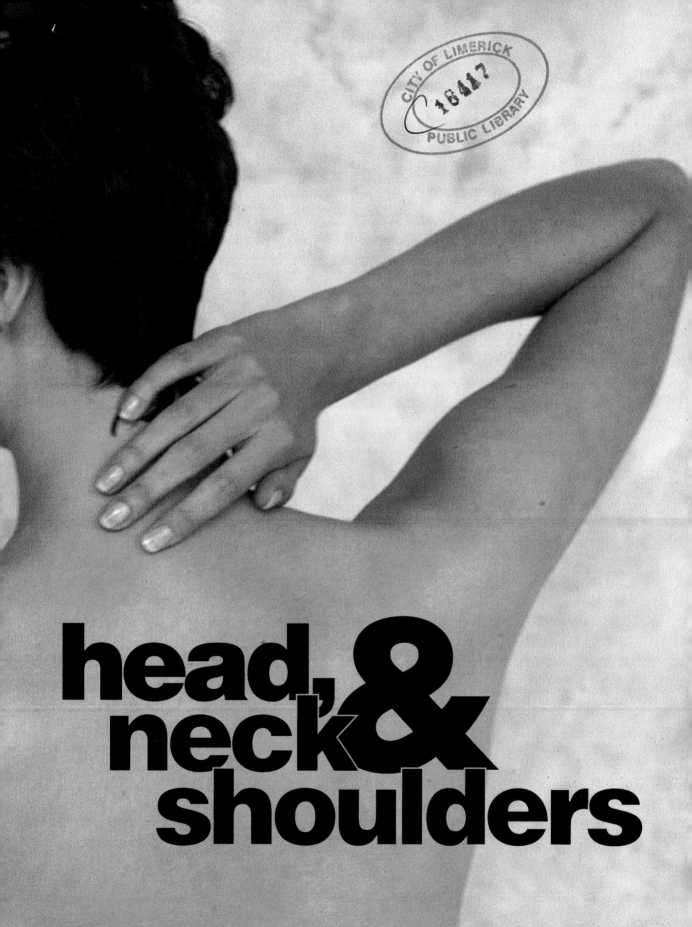

head,&
neck&
shoulders

accumulated stress, tension and poor posture can create painful, distorted shoulders and a stiff neck. In fact, the whole shoulder and neck area tends to be a prime trouble spot, so regular massage to this part of the body can be of great benefit. Incorrect posture is the main cause of misalignment that can lead to painful ligaments and joints.

Our natural response to stress does not help – we tend to hunch our neck and shoulders defensively against our problems, creating yet more postural faults. Incorrect posture will strain and stretch the upper back muscles, neck and shoulders, and allow the stomach muscles to lose their tone and strength. As a result, the diaphragm is weakened and breathing becomes shallow. Poor posture can create many tiresome health problems, including digestive disorders, breathing difficulties, and, because the muscles at the top of the back merge with the neck and support the head, migraine, headache and eye strain. All these risks prove that good posture is worth working towards. It has even been clinically proven that those people with poor posture are more susceptible to suffering from depression.

Massage can play an important role in helping to correct postural faults, as stimulating the muscles around the head, neck and shoulders will relax the chest and release the neck away from the shoulders, helping to restore correct body alignment.

Another benefit of neck and shoulder massage is that the front of the chest between the shoulders (the thoracic cavity) is where all the waste products of the body, cleansed by the lymph fluid, finally drain away. It is where the lymph fluid is returned to the circulation through veins in the upper chest, so regular massage assists this vital process.

---

note

All the full massage sequences in this book are based on a massage being given while the recipient is lying down on the floor, on a futon-style bed or a hard mattress, unless otherwise indicated.

Take care not to work too deeply and too quickly on the neck and shoulders – this area needs to be approached slowly and gently to avoid pain. Build pressure gradually, working up to deep prolonged squeezing, kneading and friction strokes to help rid the area of acute tension spots, which can be felt as hard knots of muscle.

You can massage the neck and shoulders when your partner is lying down as a part of the full massage, or use it as a separate sequence. Alternatively, massage this area with your partner in an upright position, which makes it easier to locate the areas of strain and assess the extent of stiffness.

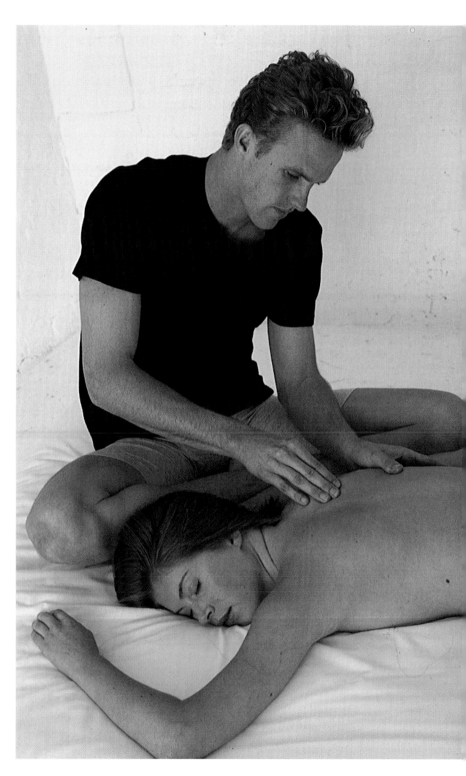

35

the full body massage stage 1

Ask your partner to lie on their back and cover their legs and torso with a towel, unless it is warm enough to massage without one.

1 Kneel behind your partner's head. Rest your hands either side of the front of the chest over the pectoral muscles, fingers pointing towards each other.

2 In one continuous movement, pull the hands away from each other and stroke them across the top of the chest up to the tops of the arms, around the arms, onto the back of the upper shoulders and up to the top of the neck. Repeat this movement as often as you like, stretching the neck gently as your hands sweep up the back of the neck into the hairline.

3 Place one hand at the base of the neck and sweep it up into the hairline. Now quickly place your other hand at the base of the neck as the first hand lets go of the top of the neck (below). Repeat the movement and alternate your hands. Ask your partner to relax so that the full weight of their head rests in your hands.

4 Using your left hand to support the weight of your partner's head, gently turn it to the left. Rest your hand on the floor and don't try to hold your partner's head up (below left). Use your right hand to stroke across their chest, over and around their shoulder and up the neck on the right hand side of their body. Pause, then slide the hand down the neck using the web of the index finger and thumb, and move along the top of the shoulder and off. Repeat the whole sequence from the beginning.

5 Change hands, move your partner's head carefully to the right side and repeat the sequence with your left hand on their left side.

6 For a gentle neck stretch, support your partner's head in your left hand while you place your right hand on their right shoulder (below right). Use your right hand to hold the shoulder down while you gently move their head to the side so that their left ear moves towards their left shoulder. This is a sideways move, so don't push the head forward while doing it. Hold the position for a few seconds before guiding the head back into the central position. Change hands and repeat the stretch on the other side. Avoid using friction at the top point of the shoulders because it will cause pain.

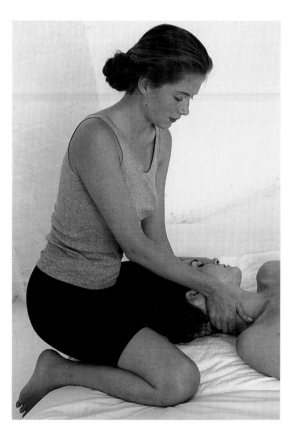

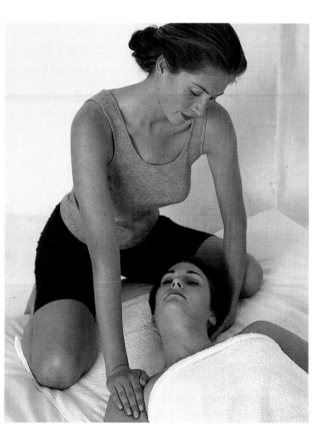

quick pick-me-ups

Neck and shoulder stiffness has many causes, including sleeping awkwardly; working hunched over a desk; anxiety; stress; sudden jarring and muscle strain. Just ten minutes of 'spot' neck and shoulder massage can give instant relief. Give a friend, partner or workmate a treat with this quick massage, which is also excellent for tiredness and hangovers, as well as general tension.

Ask your partner to sit on a chair that provides good back support. They should sit upright, with head and neck as relaxed as possible. Their feet should be flat on the floor (rest them on a book if necessary). Alternatively, have them straddle a chair, leaning forward onto cushions. They do not have to remove their clothes for this massage.

1 Stand behind them. Rest your hands on your partner's shoulders and squeeze their upper shoulder muscles. Use your body weight to lean into the movement, pressing your thumbs down and circling in tiny movements up either side of the spine towards the neck.

2 Continue with thumb circling, working in the space between the spine and shoulder blades, moving continuously over the back.

3 Slide your hands outwards onto the tops of your partner's arms, squeeze and release as you slip your hands downwards to cover the whole upper arm area with firm squeezing movements (right).

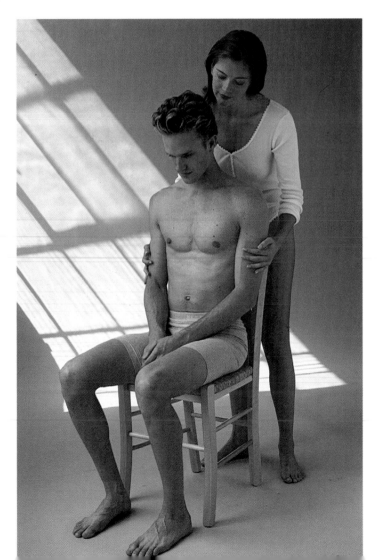

4 If your partner is sitting upright, place your right hand across the front of their chest and your left hand on the upper back. If they are straddling a chair, there is no need to place an arm across the front of the body. Keeping your left hand flat against the body, make big rubbing circular movements over the upper back to stimulate circulation and warm the muscles.

5 Slide your left hand up to rest gently on the base of their neck. Ask them to relax forwards so that they are resting their forehead in your right hand (below). Keep your fingers to the left of their neck, your open thumb to the right. Squeeze and release with fingers and thumb, working up the neck to the base of the skull. If your partner is straddled over the chair, rest their head on a cushion while the neck is worked on. Repeat from the other side if necessary.

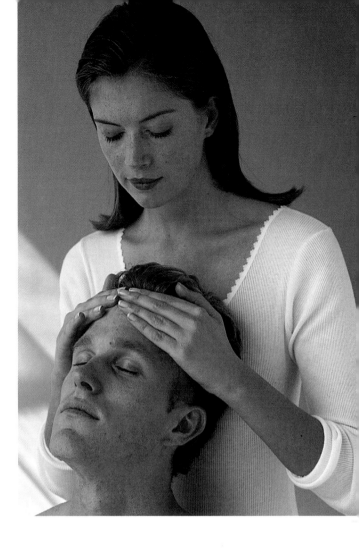

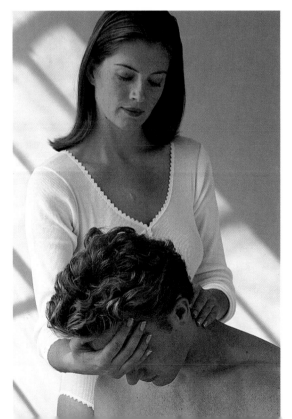

6 Whether your partner is sitting upright or leaning forward, stand behind them again and let them lean slightly backwards to rest their head against you (above). Place your flat hands over their forehead, fingers pointing towards each other. Now, massage in deep, firm and circular movements, sliding your hands apart and back across their forehead into the scalp.

7 To finish, move to the front of your partner and lightly brush your hands down their arms and legs to the feet, then lean your body weight onto their feet with your hands to 'ground' them again.

diy massage

When your shoulders and neck feel stiff, just sit down, relax, and follow these three massage moves:

1 Reach across to the right side of your shoulders with your left hand. Place your fingers over the shoulder, press your fingers into the muscles that lie behind the ridge of the shoulders as you squeeze the heel of your hand over the front muscles (below). Use firm pressure to help break up muscle tension. Now swap sides and use your right hand on the left side of your shoulders.

2 Place your right hand on the back of your head. Use your thumb to massage the right side of your neck by pressing the ball of your thumb under the bony ledge that follows the hair line from behind the ear to the back of the head (right). Press and rotate using small, firm movements. Then change hands and work the left side of the neck with your left thumb.

3 Release any remaining tension using the above stroke and stimulate your neck and shoulder area by using your right hand to 'chop' up the right side of your neck. Keep your hand flat and use the edge of the little finger in tiny, bouncing, chopping movements, up and down the neck. Then swap hands and work the left side of the neck.

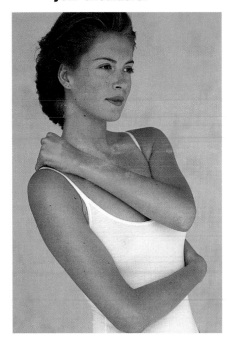

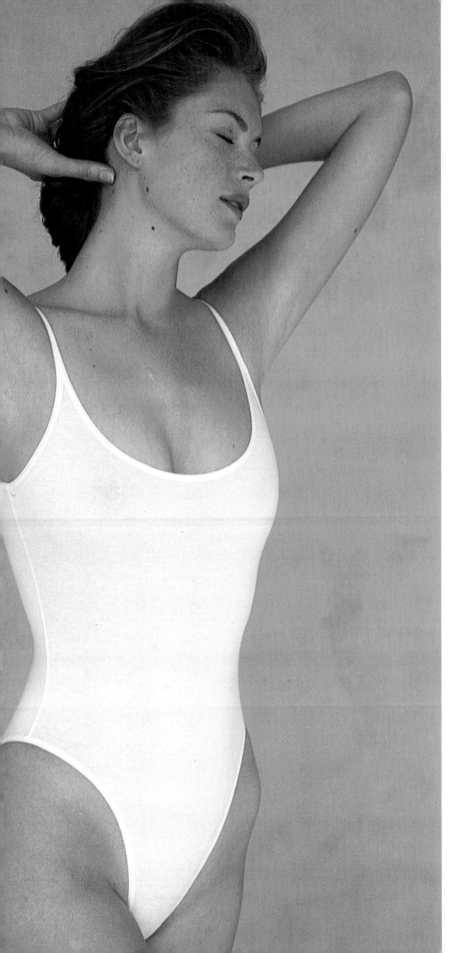

treating aches and pains

When taking a shower, give yourself a hydro massage and help to unlease tension by training a warm shower jet around the back of your neck and shoulders.

•

Self-help for an aching neck: put two tennis balls into a sock and knot the end. Lie down with the sock placed at the top of your neck, just below the base of your skull, so that each tennis ball rests either side of your spinal column. Relax in this position for about five minutes.

•

Help yourself to avoid unnecessary neck and shoulder strain by not wearing high heels every day and by avoiding carrying a heavy bag on one shoulder. If you do have to carry a heavy bag, keep switching it from shoulder to shoulder and wear the strap of your bag diagonally across your upper body.

the face

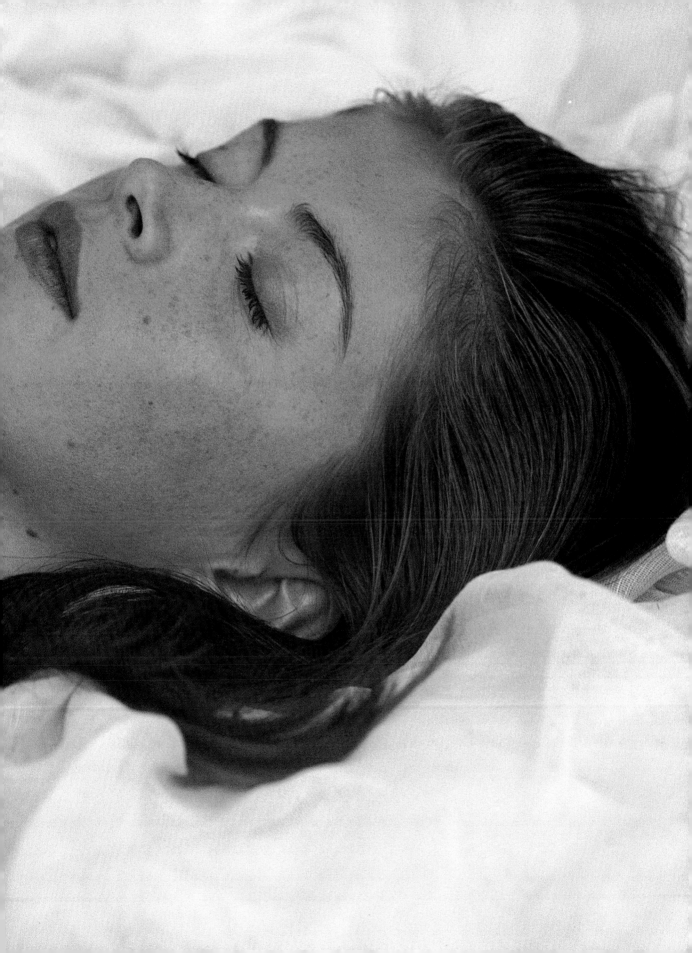

aregular facial massage will improve your skin tone and leave you feeling calm and relaxed, while a daily facial massage will give even more healthy returns – stimulated circulation, toned muscles and a glowing complexion.

When stressed, we often tense our facial muscles so as not to reveal our real feelings, so it is no surprise that this highly mobile area of the body is extremely prone to storing tension.

Tension is usually revealed in the face by a tightness in the jaw, forehead and mouth, and by a rigid expression showing worry and depression lines. The masseter, or chewing muscle, that links the jaw with the temporo-mandibular joint just in front of the ear is often prone to extreme tension, particularly in people who grip their jaw or grind their teeth – both of these unconscious actions are sure signs of stress. Massaging the face can ease away tiredness, facial tension and eyestrain, and even help alleviate headaches and sinus congestion. In fact, a face massage alone will have a relaxing and calming effect, not just on the face, but on the whole body.

The touch tactics of massage will smooth away minor stress lines and help drain excess lymph fluid and wastes that can cause puffy skin. Bags under the eyes can also sometimes benefit from acupressure applied to key points on the face, which also helps to relieve sinus congestion.

When massaging the face your movements should be firm, especially over the bony sinus areas on the cheekbones. Direct your strokes upward and outwards, following the main lines of facial expression. Always use a cream or oil to help your fingers glide over the skin and avoid dragging it. Take care not to pull, squeeze or pinch sensitive facial skin, especially around the eyes. It's also best to avoid working directly on the eyelids as they are especially sensitive. The best position for your partner to be in to receive a facial massage is lying down on a comfortable surface such as a futon. This will relieve the pull of gravity on the delicate facial tissues.

the full body massage stage 2

Touching the face is an intimate thing to do, so treat it with awareness and sensitivity. Check if your partner is wearing contact lenses, as these should be removed, along with any jewellery. Stand behind your partner's head and take it in your hands, holding it gently to give them time to relax and become familiar with your touch before you begin the massage.

1 Place your thumbs together in the centre of the forehead. Slide them apart across the forehead and up to the hairline (below). Keep repeating this action until you have covered the entire forehead, moving across to the ears with soft sliding strokes. Avoid pressing too hard or you will drag the skin.

2 Use your thumbs to slide firmly across the brow bone above the eyes and continue until you reach the edge of the face.

3 Move your thumbs to the under-eye area. Working along the eye socket bone, sweep your thumbs from the inner corners of the eyes, nearest the nose, massaging outwards and across, to follow the curve of the cheekbones.

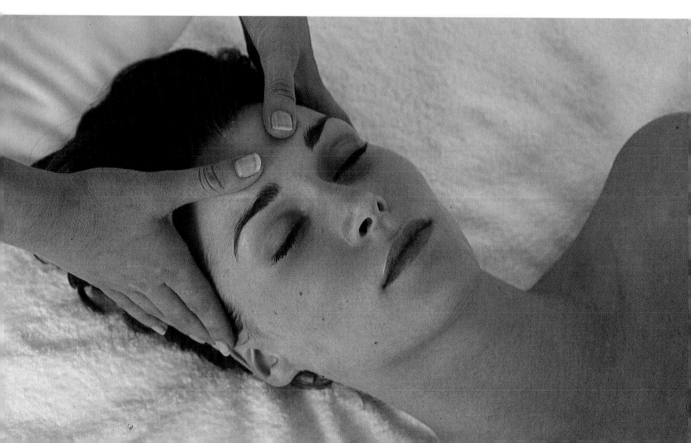

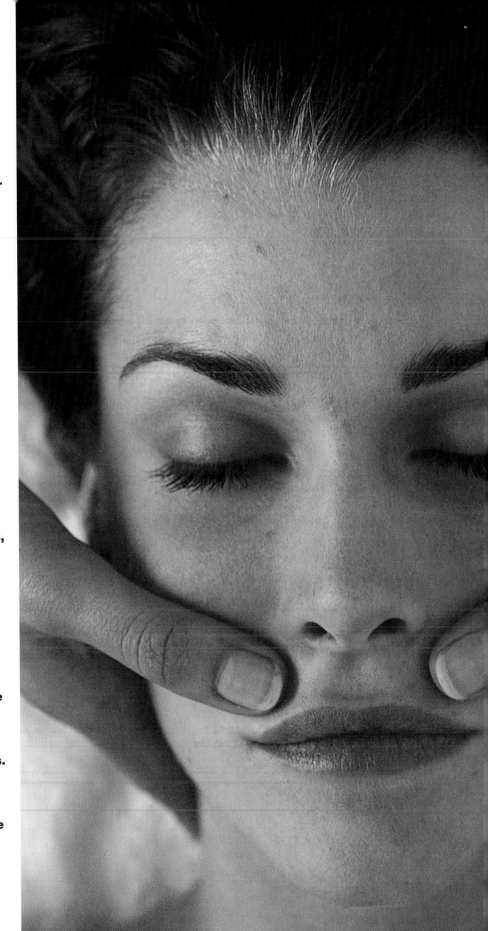

4 Place your thumbs over the top lip so that they meet just under your partner's nose. Now slide them apart moving across the top lip and downwards (right). Repeat this movement under the bottom lip, sliding your thumbs from the centre of the chin outwards.

5 To massage the jawline, place your thumbs on top of the chin and your fingers under the jaw. Gently squeeze along the jaw from the centre outwards, using a kneading action to work against the bone.

6 Place your fingers behind the ears and the heels of your hands in front of the ears so that you enclose your partner's ears in the palms of your hands. Now gently stretch the ears, pulling them downwards. Repeat this a couple of times.

7 Give the whole outer ear area a massage by lightly squeezing the lobe of the ears between index fingers and thumbs, squeezing and circling fingers and thumbs in small movements all around the ear lobes and up around the outer rim of the ears. This can sometimes result in a warm sensation in the ears.

Note: In Chinese medicine the ears have different points that correspond to all the organs in the body, therefore they believe that ear massage and performing acupressure on the ear is an important part of health care.

8 Move your fingers up above the ears and into the hairline, working over the scalp with deep 'shampooing' movements. Concentrate on the crown of the head and the point at the back of the head where the skull joins the neck, massaging with tense fingers for a more vigorous and firm effect. However, don't scrub at the head. Work on, using just the pads of the fingers in controlled, firm and circular movements. You should feel the scalp move back and forth. As so much tension is stored in the scalp, a regular massage can be very beneficial. It is also valuable in treating the many scalp and hair disorders that are triggered by stress.

9 To finish, comb your fingers through your partner's hair, giving the roots a very gentle pull at the end of each stroking movement, to release tension (right). **This has a soothing effect and can also feel very sensual too.**

Note: As you will probably be using a lubricating massage oil, check that your partner is happy to have this taken up into the hair. Although scalp massage is an important part of face massage, it can be omitted if your partner does not want to be left with oily hair at the end of the session.

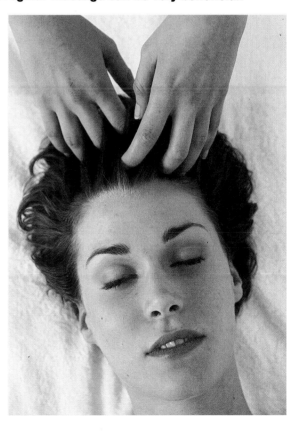

diy massage

These simple DIY massage moves can be performed at any time to help soothe a headache or relieve tiredness.

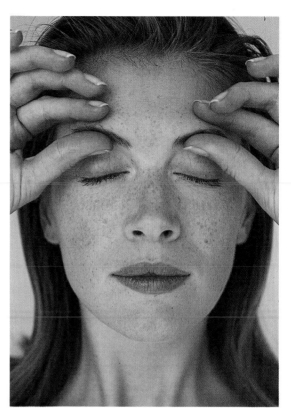

1 Starting from the centre of your eyebrows, sweep fingers up and over your forehead and out to the hairline.

2 Using thumb and fingers gently pinch along the browbone over your eyebrows, working from the centre outwards (above right). **This acts on acupressure points and has a stimulating, reviving effect.**

3 Using your first two fingertips, press under the cheekbones, following the curve of your lower eye socket line, working into the skin, pressing, holding and releasing as you move your fingers along from the nose outwards towards your ears.

relieving headaches

To soothe a headache, add a drop of lavender oil to a carrier oil and massage over your forehead and temples. The forehead is the most common site in which to experience all the pain of a headache, so firm, soothing strokes over this area will help the flow of blood and prevent congestion.

•

To ease sinus congestion, add a drop of marjoram essential oil to a carrier oil, and massage.

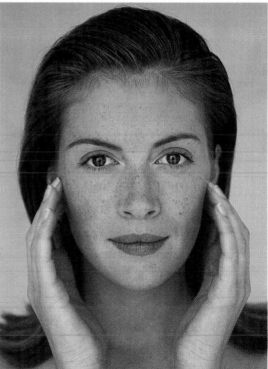

4 For facial tension use your fingertips to massage your cheeks, pressing into the soft, fleshy part of your cheeks and feeling the underlying bone structure (right). Use small, firm circular movements to work the muscles that lie under the cheekbones.

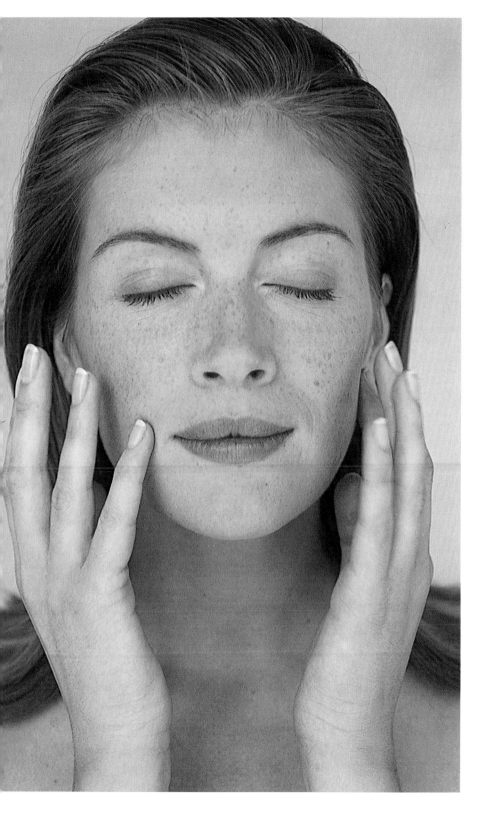

5 Place your fingers over the chin, thumbs under the jawline, and pinch along the jaw, working from the centre outwards.

6 To waken and stimulate your face, drum your fingertips lightly and quickly all over your face, keeping your eyelids closed (left).

skin rebalancers

Treat dry, sensitive complexions with two drops of rose and two drops of camomile essence in a carrier oil such as jojoba or avocado.

•

Massage oily skin with lavender essence mixed with a carrier oil, then wipe away any excess using a tissue.

•

Two drops of neroli essence mixed with two drops of lavender in a carrier oil will help improve blemishes and acne.

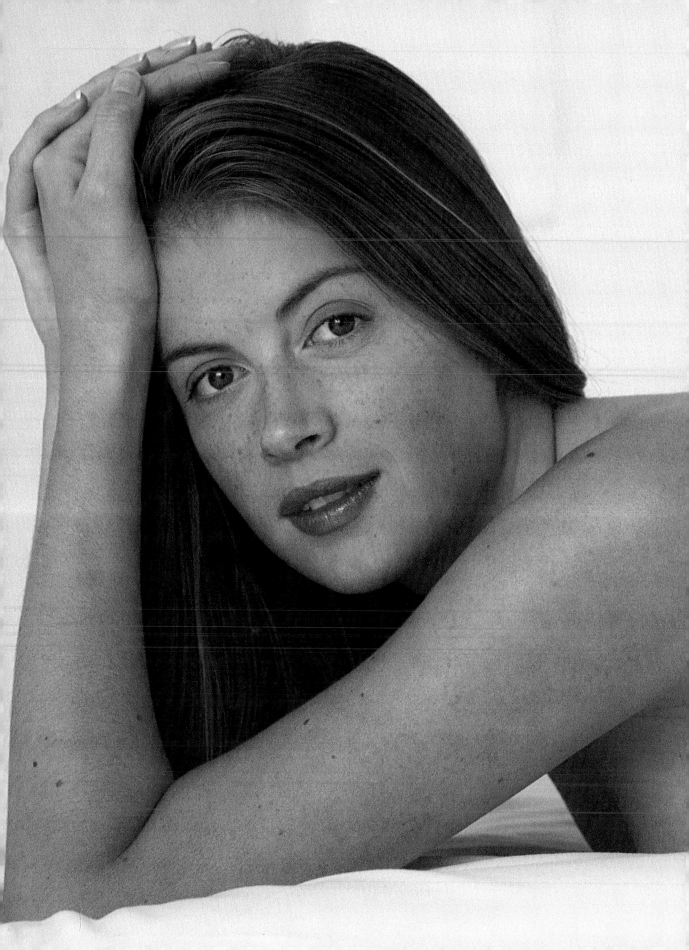

the back

the back is the largest single area of the body, and so deserves a little extra time and attention during a full massage.

The back also contains some of the largest muscles in the body, many of which connect the spine to the limbs. Thirty-one pairs of spinal nerves branch out over the back from the shoulders to the waist. These are connected to all the internal organs, while other, longer nerve branches radiate out to the limbs. One of the largest back muscles is the trapezius, a flat muscle that extends from the base of the skull to the lower region of the spine and connects to the shoulder-blade – the trapezius is often a site of tension, causing discomfort in the neck, shoulder and upper back.

According to UK government health statistics, one in twenty people consult their doctor each year with back problems. It is also the largest cause of absenteeism from work.

Whilst some backaches can be caused by internal problems like kidney infection or constipation, over 95 per cent of all back pain is caused by musculo/skeletal disorders. A professional massage can help to treat severe backache, but regular home massages can help to ease niggling aches and pains too. In many cases massage will prevent backache from worsening and developing into a more serious problem.

Because of the complex nerve structure in the back which spreads to every other part of the body, a sense of total release and well-being can be felt after a back massage. Of course it is physically impossible to give yourself a proper back massage, so lie back, relax and let a friend do the work for you.

the full body massage stage 3

With your partner lying on their front, place a pillow under the body to support and lift the affected area.

1 Kneel beside your partner, knees approximately level with their hips, facing towards their head (right above). **Begin with effleurage strokes (see pages 24-26) working from the base of the spine up to the top of the shoulders. Apply firm pressure on the upward stroke and when you reach the top of the shoulders, slide your fingers over the tops of the shoulders, pause to squeeze and lift the muscle then release the pressure and let your hands trail lightly back down the body to the starting point. Repeat often, making sure you cover the whole of the back.**

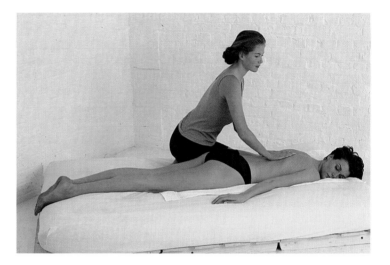

2 Work all over the back in circular effleurage strokes. This can be repeated for as long as you like – the idea is to warm your partner's muscles and stimulate their circulation. The repetitive rhythm of the strokes will also help your partner to relax.

3 When you are ready, move to face the top of the body and kneel above your partner's head (right below). Repeat the first long, sweeping effleurage stroke from the top of the spine down to the buttocks and back again. But this time maintain firm pressure on both the upward and downward strokes. Repeat.

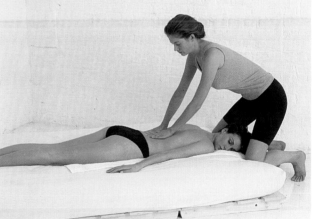

4 Position your thumbs either side of the spine, lean your weight into them and slide down your partner's back in one long smooth movement. Release the pressure and trail your hands back to the top of the spine where you can repeat.

5 Place your flat hands over your partner's shoulder blades. Moving your right hand, lean your weight into the heel of your hand and sweep it upwards to the top of the spine, then across their shoulders on your right and down onto the top of the arm, pushing downwards to stretch and widen the shoulders. As you lift your right hand off their body, move your left hand over the other side of their body, which is on your left side, repeating the stroke. Repeat this pattern, alternating your hands.

6 Move back to the side of the body and, starting at the base of the spine, stroke both hands up the back using your thumbs to exert extra pressure either side of the spine (below). Slide your hands gently back to the base of the spine and repeat the process.

7 Turn to face the side of your partner's body and begin working with petrissage strokes (see pages 26-28). You should be kneeling for this stroke (opposite above). Keep your knees apart and your back straight, lean forward from the hips and do not twist or strain your own body. Use both hands to squeeze and knead the muscles that run from the spine out across the body. Work from the right of the spine outwards starting from the base of the back and moving up to the shoulder blade, squeezing and kneading.

This stroke feels especially good in the soft fleshy waist area above the pelvis. Move to the right side of your partner to repeat the move on the left hand side of the body.

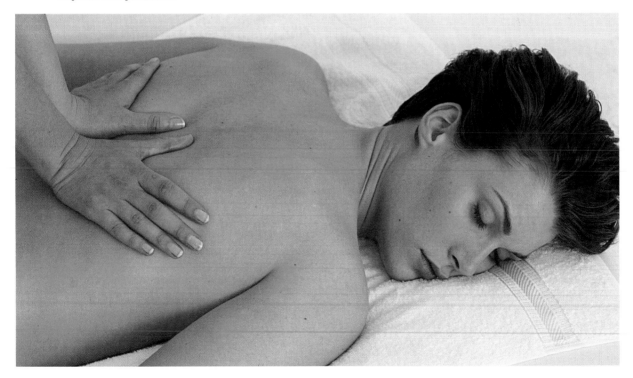

8 Re-position yourself so that you turn and face up towards your partner's head, your knees together (right below). At this point make sure that your partner's arms are positioned correctly – they should be out to the sides of their body in an 'arrow' position. Do not allow their arms to be placed above the line of their shoulders otherwise they will distort their shoulders and reduce the effect of the shoulder massage you are about to give them. Their face should be turned away from the shoulder you are working on. Use both of your hands alternately to push and pull in petrissage strokes over the shoulder area. Use the whole of your hands, including your fingertips, to work into the muscle fibre. As you let go with one hand, push down with the other to maintain a continuous movement over one shoulder. Change sides and work on the other side of the body.

9 Deepen the massage by moving on to friction strokes (see pages 28-29). Use your thumbs to make large circular movements all around the shoulder blades, working from the sides inwards and then up the spine onto the neck.

10 Concentrate on any tight spots by working more intensely on these areas. Press down with the pad of your thumb, maintain the pressure and then make tiny circular movements. Ask your partner to breathe out as you press down. Check to see if any pain is felt when you apply pressure.

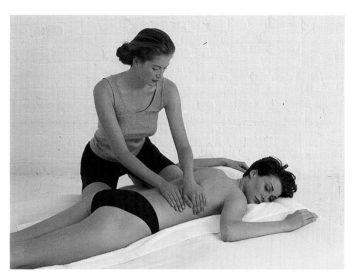

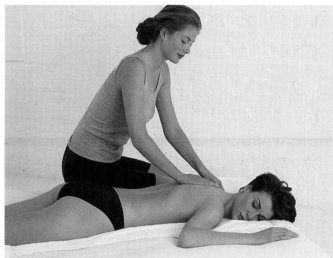

11 Finish with thumb rolling. Change position so that you are kneeling above your partner's head. Working in the space diagonally between the spine and the shoulder blade, use the length of your thumb to lean in and slide through that space. Work with one thumb, and follow it immediately with the other. This action is carried out quickly and gives your partner the impression of your thumbs rolling over the skin.

quick pick-me-ups

Tapotement (see pages 29-31) can be used at the end of the whole back massage sequence, or it can be used as a stimulating quick pick-me-up on its own. Warm and prepare the back first with five minutes of effleurage strokes (see pages 24-26). Tapotement is very invigorating, but should not hurt. If your partner has extra sensitive skin, place a thin towel on their back to reduce stinging.

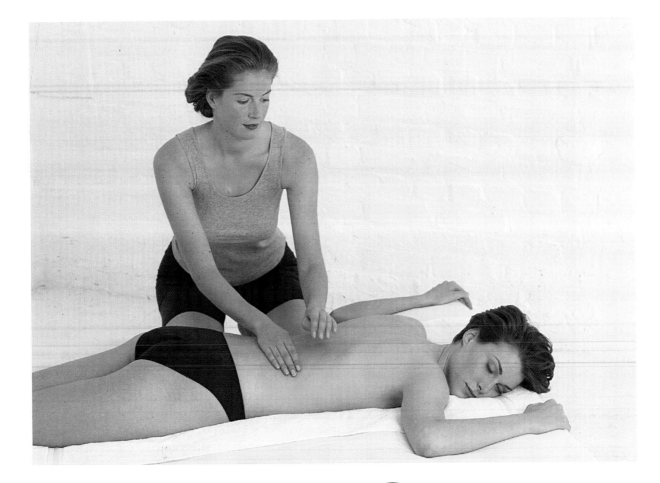

1 Stand or kneel to one side of your partner's body and drum your cupped hands all over their back (above).

2 Curl your hands into fists, and lightly but firmly drum them over the fleshy areas of the buttocks and thighs.

back problems

● **mid backache** Aching in the mid back is often caused by tightness in the vertical bands of muscle on either side of the spine. You will find that slow, gliding strokes over the area of pain will be soothing. Pushing across the spinal muscles with the heels of your hands from one side of your spine out across that half of the back will comfort the area.

● **lower backache** A very common site for tension, and therefore pain. Help to relieve aching in this area with rhythmic circling movements followed by generous kneading. This will work the muscles slowly and thoroughly.

● **sciatica** Sciatica is a sharp, shooting pain in the legs, buttocks and back. It usually affects only one side of the body and is sometimes accompanied by tingling in the leg or foot. It is caused by pressure on the sciatic nerve. If the pain is persistent and severe, and/or is felt on both sides of the body, get help from a doctor or osteopath. Most sciatica cases will heal themselves in time. Meanwhile, plenty of rest and regular gentle massage will help. Try this technique: press down with the heels of your hands on either side of the spine, just above the buttocks, with fingers pointing outwards, then gradually slide your hands away from each other out across the buttocks. Return and repeat the process several times. You can also knead the entire buttock area, but stop if this becomes painful.

backache soothers

Marjoram essence mixed with a carrier oil will help to ease muscular pains and painful joints.

●

Rosemary is a refreshing, stimulating essential oil; mixed with a carrier oil it also helps soothe muscular aches.

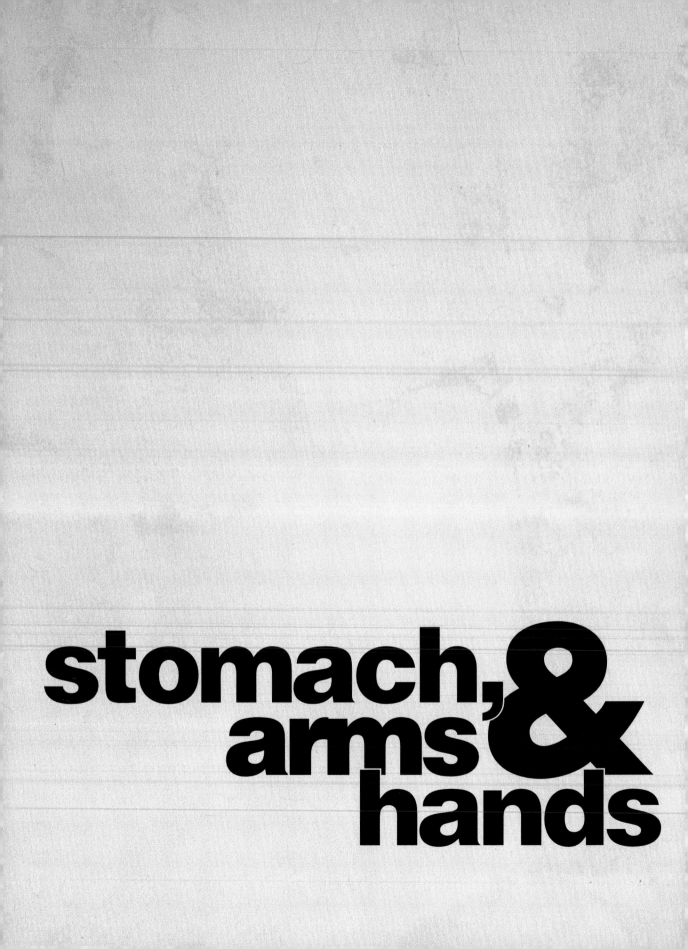

stomach,&
arms'&
hands

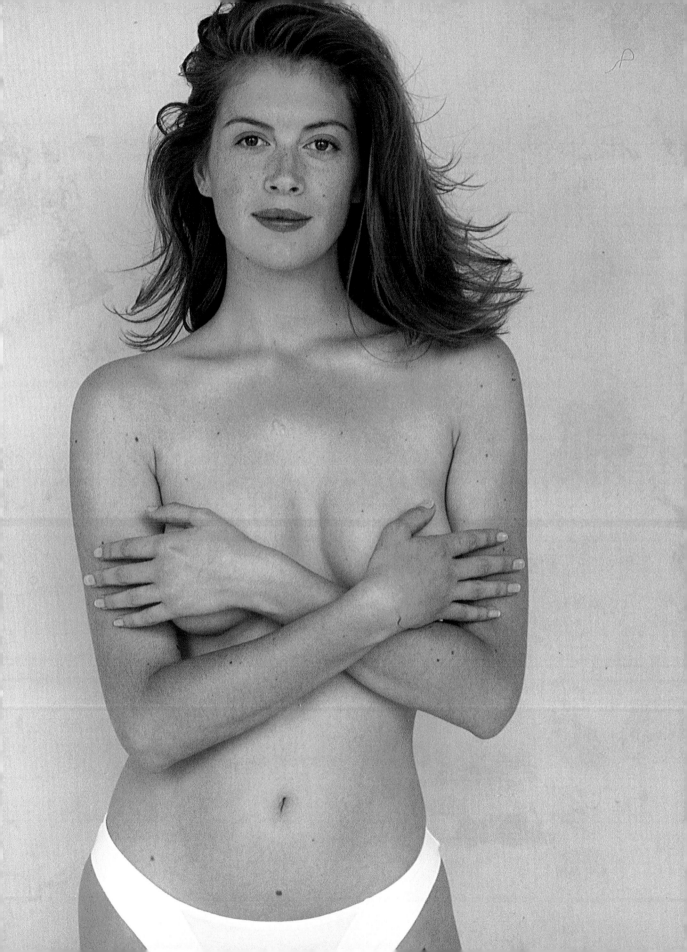

stomach

The stomach is our centre of gravity, but it is often distorted by restrictive clothing and poor posture. Stomach tension can inhibit natural breathing and reduce energy levels. In addition, any weakness in the abdominal region will lead to an instability of the lumbar spine, and therefore a tendency to place too much strain on the lumbar muscles.

The digestive system and the digestive organs – the liver, gall bladder and pancreas – are all affected by the condition of the stomach muscles and other tissues surrounding them. Massage is therefore an excellent therapy for many digestive disorders because it can help to relax and/or strengthen the abdominal muscles. It will also stimulate a sluggish digestive system, preventing or relieving bloating and constipation. Massage work over the stomach can also promote secretion of enzymes by the digestive glands and so aid digestion, while increased blood flow to the abdomen will improve the assimilation of nutrients into the bloodstream. After a meal, allow two hours to pass before being massaged.

arms & hands

The muscles and joints of the shoulder allow a great freedom and variety of movement in this area, but many people experience tension in these hardworking muscles, particularly after physical activity. The biceps muscle in the upper arm is also prone to strain through heavy manual activity. The flexor muscles in the forearm can be protected from strain through massage, which will reduce any shortening of the muscles and release tension from the hands. Tension can build up gradually and imperceptibly in the fingers and wrists. This can be due to anxiety and worry, or to performing tasks that require a great deal of manual dexterity and control. Stiffness in the finger joints can be caused by poor circulation or arthritis, while chilblains, caused by a restricted blood flow, may afflict fingers in cold weather. Hands are subjected to daily physical abuse and deserve plenty of care to keep them looking and feeling healthy. The thousands of sensitive nerve endings in the palms and fingertips make hands very receptive to a massage, which will increase their dexterity.

the full body massage stage 4

● stomach

Ask your partner to lie on their back, hands relaxed at their sides or above their head, palms up. They may find it more comfortable to bend their knees, to help relax the abdominal muscles.

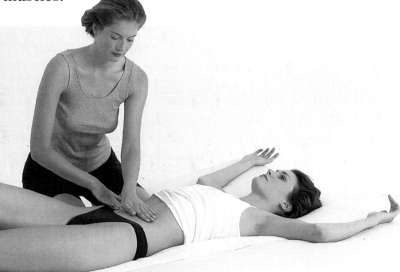

1 Begin by placing yourself to the right of your partner's body and position your left hand on the left side of their stomach, your right hand resting behind your left one (right). Now work in clockwise circles around the stomach, following an area of the digestive system. You can use quite a firm pressure for this.

2 Using petrissage strokes, (see pages 26-28) knead the skin and underlying muscles on the left hand side of the body around the soft stomach area (right).

3 Change sides and repeat the process.

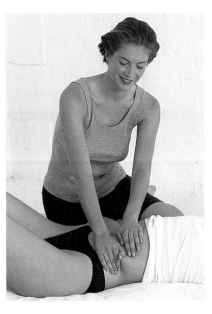

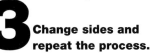

4 Slide your thumbs firmly under and along the ribcage, making sure your partner's breathing is relaxed.

the solar plexus

Find your solar plexus, which is positioned 5cm (2in) below your breastbone: it is believed to be the site of our intuition. Massage in this area is supposed to help in the development of psychic powers and it should also give the body extra energy in times of stress.

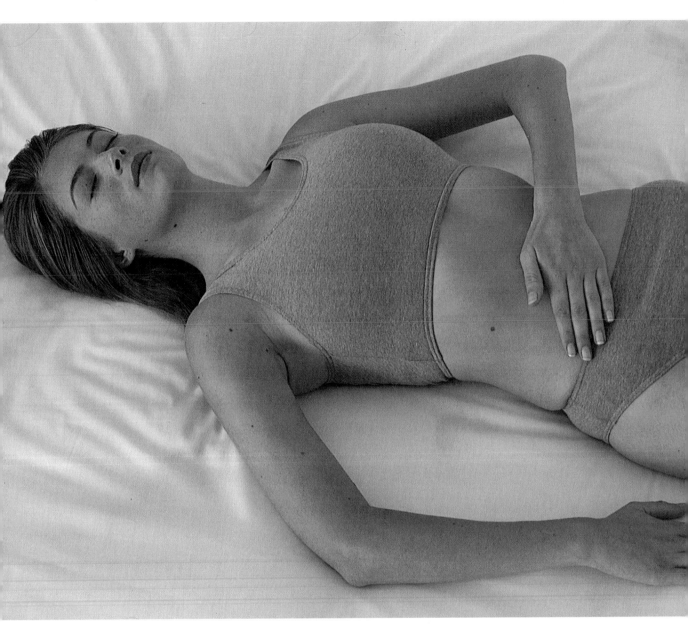

diy massage

● stomach

To help relieve period pains and a bloated, sluggish digestive system, lie on your back, knees bent, and use one hand to rub your tummy in circular, clockwise movements. You can press quite firmly.

the full body massage stage 5

● arms

Encourage your partner to make their whole arm and hand go limp, as the arms and hands are often the most difficult parts to 'let go'.

1 Hold their right arm at the wrist with your right hand and use your left hand to stroke firmly up the front of the arm to the shoulder and back down the underside of the arm to the wrist (right).

2 Still holding the wrist with your right hand, slide your left hand towards their inner elbow, then twist your hands so that your fingers slip lower beneath their forearm, and slide your hand back down to the wrist (below). **Your fingers and thumb should exert firm pressure on the upward and downward strokes.**

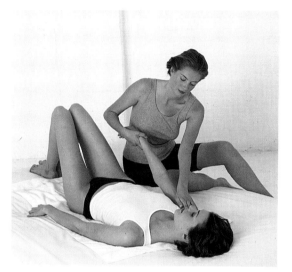

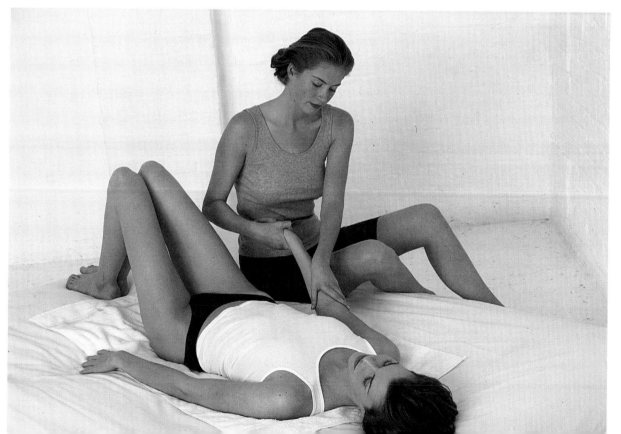

3 Move your supporting hand to their elbow and use the other hand to squeeze along their upper arm (right). **Move fingers and thumb together in a kneading action.**

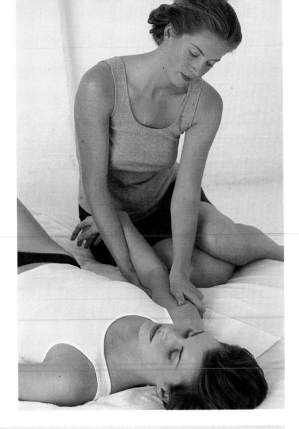

4 Position yourself so that you are kneeling by their shoulder. Lift up the arm nearest to you so that it leans against you; your partner should let their whole arm relax so that it bends naturally at the elbow with the forearm falling forwards onto their own body (right below). Wrap your hands around their upper arm by the crease of their elbow: your thumbs should be in the elbow crease, fingers underneath the arm. Now squeeze and slowly slide your hands down from the elbow crease to the armpit. Relax, release the pressure and glide your hands back to the starting point to repeat the move.

5 Place your partner's arm above their head, letting it bend naturally at the elbow and leaving it to lie flat and relaxed above their heads in a comfortable position. Hold your partner's wrist with one hand while you place your other hand flat over their pectoral muscle just above their breast. Lean in with your weight and slide your hand over the pectoral muscle and up, just onto the top of the arm. Repeat this short stroke several times.

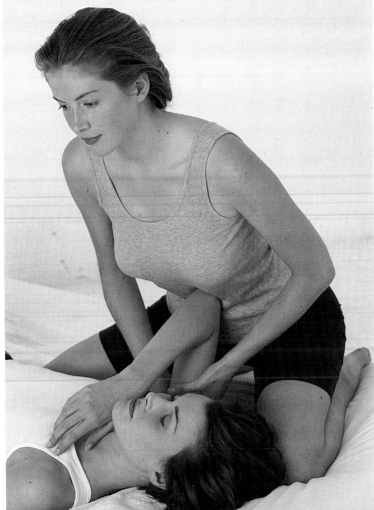

● hands

Keep the skin on your hands in great condition by applying a hand cream after every hand wash. You can take the opportunity to give yourself a quick DIY hand massage too.

1 Hold your partner's right hand, resting their palm on the fingers of both your hands (right). **Circle your thumbs over the back of their hands in small, circular movements, using the underlying bones as a guideline.**

2 Turn the hand over. Hold with your right hand and use your left thumb to circle deeply into the soft flesh at the base of their thumb (below left). **Work out across the wrist and circle around the cushioned area of the palm.**

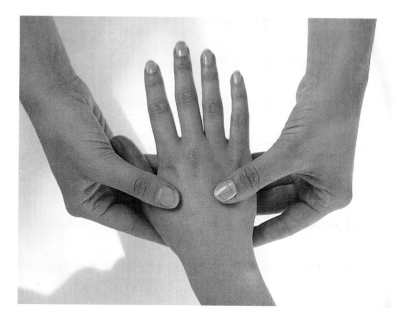

3 Turn the hand over again and hold in your left hand while you use your right hand to squeeze and pull each finger in turn (below right). **Concentrate on a gentle pulling movement as you twist your fingers around theirs, pulling and sliding upwards. Start with the thumb and work on each finger in turn.**

4 Now move to their left side and repeat the arm and hand massage sequence on their left arm.

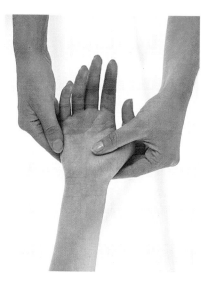

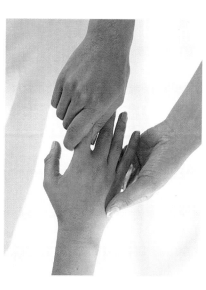

diy massage

● **arms**

1 Use your thumb and fingers to squeeze your way down your opposite arm from the shoulder to the **wrist** (below).

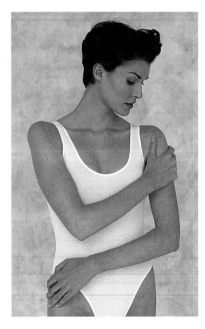

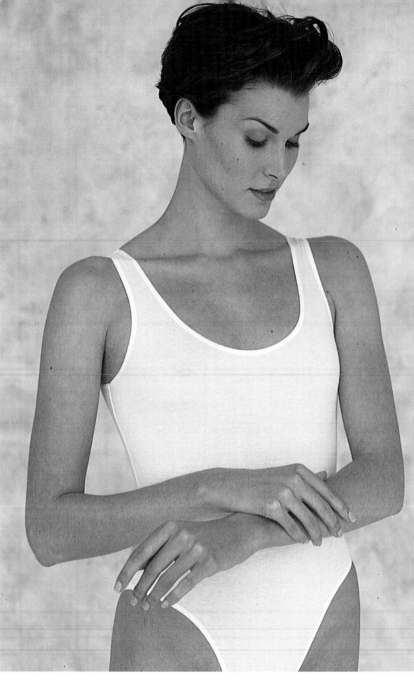

2 To exert deeper pressure, use your thumb to work the middle area of your forearm, massaging into the soft area between the bones (above right). **Press, make a tiny circle, release, and slide your thumb upwards to repeat the movement. Cover the area from wrist to elbow.**

● **hands**

1 Use your thumb and fingers to squeeze your way down your opposite arm from the shoulder to the wrist.

2 Squeeze and gently pull each finger in turn, starting with the thumb.

quick pick-me-ups

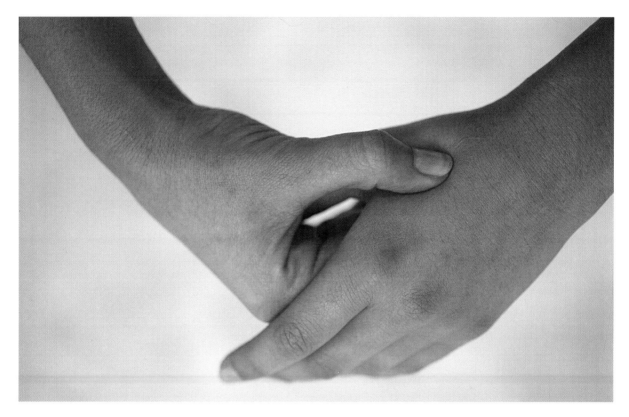

● **stiff hands** Massage around the joints of all your fingers and each thumb.

● **tired fingers** Place your hands over the desk/table as if playing the piano, then softly tap the fingertips on the table in rapid, bouncing movements. Try to keep your arms relaxed as you do this.

hand care

Soothe and nourish chapped, cracked skin with camomile or rose essential oil diluted with a carrier oil.

●

Mix up some sugar in equal proportions with sunflower oil and massage onto hands to clean stained skin.

●

Soak chapped, rough hands in a bowl of warm milk for five minutes each night.

● **headache** When you are anxious, stressed or suffering from a headache you can work the 'Eliminator' point on your hand – find it in the web of skin between your thumb and hand, just above the joint (*above*). Press here repeatedly whenever you need to relax or shake off a headache.

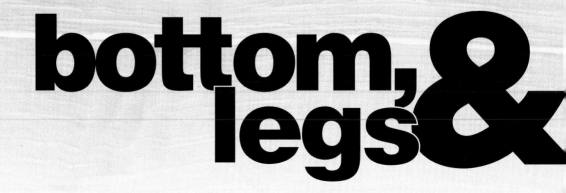

bottom, & legs &

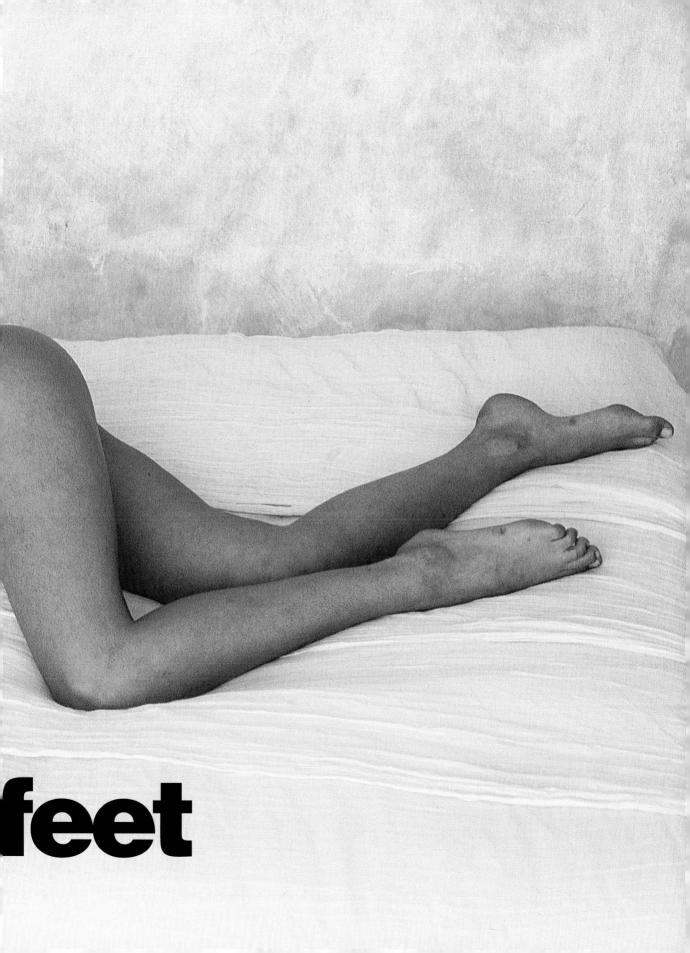

feet

because our legs and feet take the strain of our body's weight, they are often prone to aches and pains, while the bottom and thigh area is the place where cellulite can develop. Both areas can benefit from regular massage.

Cellulite, the uneven fatty phenomenon which is essentially a woman's problem, tends to accumulate around the thighs, bottom and hips. Cellulite is thought to be a build-up of fats, water and wastes in the connective skin tissues, and unfortunately it is notoriously hard to shift. Fluid retention, hormonal imbalances, poor circulation and impaired lymphatic drainage have all been identified as possible causes, while lack of exercise and an unbalanced diet can contribute to the problem. For anyone serious about dealing with their cellulite, regular massage – along with an exercise programme and healthy eating – is an essential undertaking. Luckily the soft, fleshy backs of the legs and buttocks respond very well to petrissage and tapotement strokes (see pages 26 and 29) that help the body to rid itself of waste and fight cellulite.

The sciatic nerve runs from the base of the spine down the back of the leg to the heel, so massaging the back of the leg can help to relieve tenderness in the area and can also ease stiffness in the lower back.

The muscles of the front of the legs and feet work extremely hard. They are used constantly, so are prone to stored tension which prevents force from being evenly distributed along the leg. Massaging the calf muscles can break up this tension.

The feet are made up of a complex network of twenty six small bones and a dense weave of muscles, ligaments and tendons, with thousands of nerve endings concentrated in the sole, which also acts as a shock absorber. If you're on your feet all day, extra strain is placed on the ankles and feet. Massage can help to ease this strain by promoting better circulation and reducing fluid retention. A foot massage will relax and soothe the whole body, while toning and strengthening those crucial muscles that actually support the entire body's weight.

the full body massage stage 6

● legs and buttocks

Ask your partner to lie on their front. For extra comfort you could raise and support their ankle with a small rolled-up towel. Legs should be relaxed and slightly apart, with toes naturally turning inwards.

1 **Your first position is to kneel beside your partner's ankles, facing towards their body** (right). **As you move into a stroke, kneel up and lean forwards so that you can press down more easily. This action will actually place some strain on your own thighs and buttocks, so make sure you keep your knees together and your back straight to make it easier on yourself. Begin with effleurage strokes (see pages 24-26) to oil and soothe the whole of the leg, stroking from the back of the heel up to the top of the leg. Keep your hands flat and pointing up the leg, and exert pressure only on the upward stroke.**

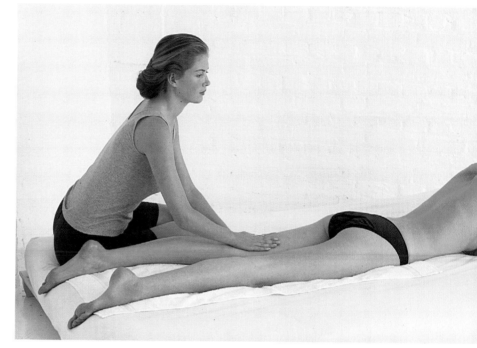

2 **Cup hands, with closed fingers, and turn them sideways, placing them over the legs to stimulate the skin over the calves in upward strokes.**

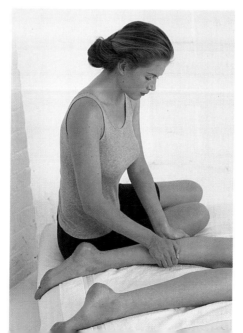

3 **Place the heels of your hands together over the top of the calf and firmly press and slide hands across the calf, away from each other** (left). **Work up to the knee over the Achilles tendon.**

4 Place hands flat against the leg, above the knee, and sweep hands up the thighs in firm effleurage strokes. Your outer hand can slide up and over the buttock but your inner hand should stop at a 'polite' point on the inner thigh!

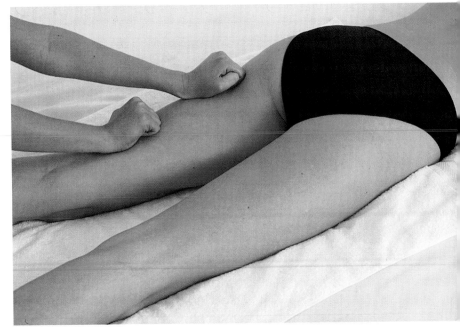

5 For deeper work on the large thigh muscles, bend fingers and press the flat middle sections of the fingers into the leg (right). Continue pressing and stroking over the whole of this area for as long as if feels right. This movement works well on stiff hamstrings and helps the body eliminate waste from the area.

6 Change your position so that you are kneeling, facing the body. Now work over the calf muscles with both hands flat on the leg, fingers and thumbs open. Wring the muscles in a backwards and forwards movement, working in opposite directions and stretching the tissue between your hands.

7 Wring the thighs with big movements using the whole of your hands on the area. Keep your fingers closed (right). As your fingers slip under your partner's thighs, lift the muscle up then let it go again.

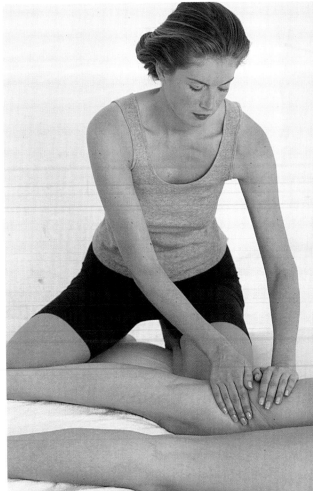

8 Move to the other side of your partner to practise firm petrissage strokes (see pages 26-28) over the buttock (below). These are best applied while you are kneeling up and over their body. Press the heel of the hand into the buttock near the sacrum, slide down and pull back. Lean your weight into your hands. Repeat with the other hand, alternating hands and maintaining a continuous movement over the whole area.

9 Ask your partner to turn onto their back. If your partner has lower back problems, place a pillow below their knees. Kneel, facing towards their body. Apply the oil in effleurage strokes covering the entire front of the leg. As there is little muscle on the shins, concentrate most of your massage work on the upper legs, above the knees. Concentrate on big, firm effleurage strokes, reaching up as far as you can.

10 Work from above the knee up the thigh with petrissage movements, lifting, pulling and kneading the muscle. However, as the bone of the thigh is nearer to the surface on the front of the leg, you should exert less pressure here than you did on the back of the leg. If your massage partner is pregnant, don't work too long or deeply on the inner thigh.

11 Turn to face your partner's leg, your own knees apart. Work around the knee using smaller wringing movements and not too much pressure. Then move your hands up and over the thigh using larger, firmer wringing movements, as used on the back of the leg.

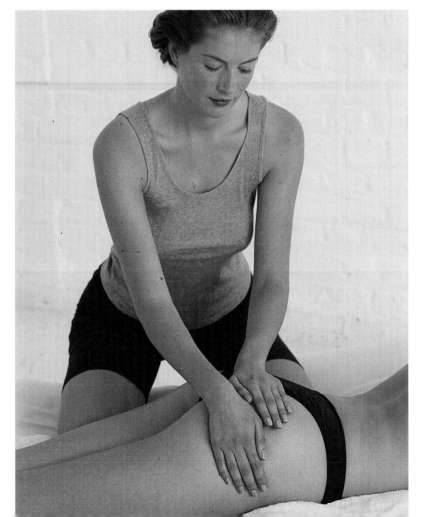

treating swollen legs

Work on 'draining' the leg to help reduce puffy tissues. Place both your hands sideways over your partner's ankle, keeping your fingers closed and your thumbs open, cupping the legs. Glide your cupped hand up the leg, pressing down firmly. Alternate with your other hand as your first hand reaches the limit of its stroke. Keep alternating hands in rhythmical strokes, working over the whole of the back of the leg.

diy massage

● legs

You can perform this DIY massage anywhere that is comfortable and relatively private, but it is both relaxing and convenient to do it in the bath. Invest in a non-slip bath mat for extra safety.

1 Bend the leg you are working on. Begin by stroking with firm, smooth effleurage movements up the back of the calf (right).

2 Squeeze and press the calf muscle using fingers and thumbs on both hands (below right).

3 Stroke from the knee up the thigh with both hands.

4 Squeeze and knead the muscles, working from the knee to the groin.

5 Use the inner edges of your flat hands to hack lightly but firmly over the fatty areas of the thigh. Finish by pummelling the same areas with your fists.

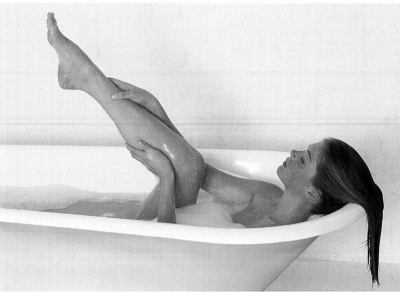

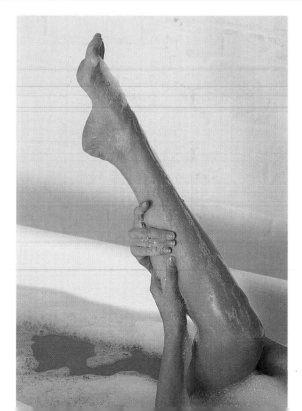

the full body massage stage 7

● feet

It will be more pleasant for your partner if you use a refreshing foot cream rather than an oil when massaging the feet. You could also cover the rest of the legs with a towel.

1 Stroke the whole of the foot gently, from toes to ankles, using both hands (right).

2 Support their heel with one hand and use the other hand to carefully rotate, stretch and flex the foot.

3 Using both hands, place your thumbs over the top of your partner's foot and massage in firm, rotating movements over the whole area, working up from the base of their toes to the ankle (right below).

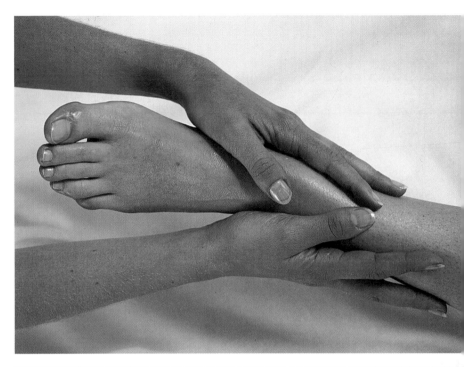

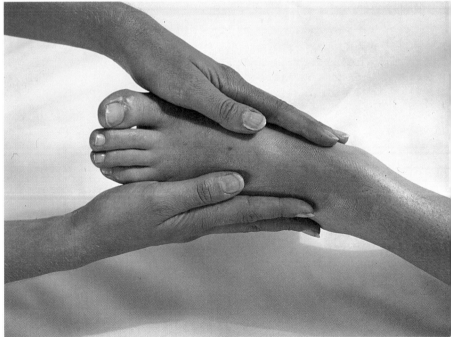

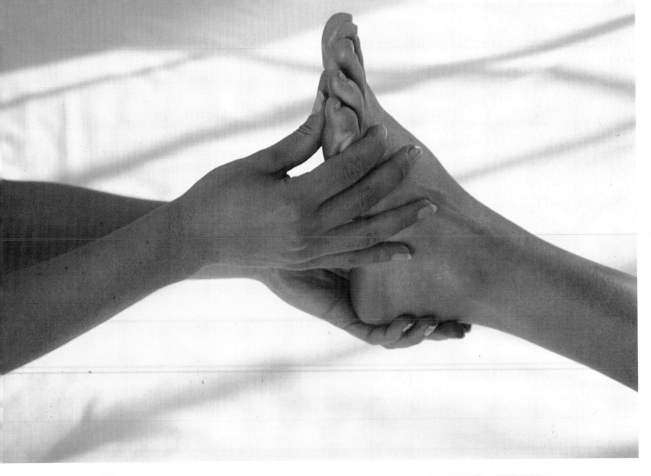

4 Support their heel with one hand while you use the thumb of your other hand to press and rotate over their sole (above). Prop their foot on your leg or a rolled up towel and take their foot in both your hands. Work up to and onto the ball of the foot and across the base of the toes, massaging with your thumbs.

5 Gently stretch and squeeze each toe by twisting and pulling your fingers over them (above right).

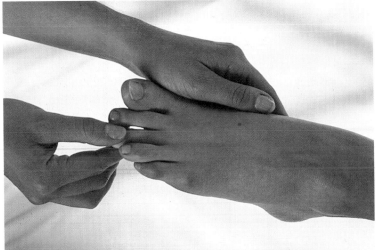

6 To finish the massage, place one of your hands on your partner's sole and the other on the top of their foot. Now slide your hands in a warm, enfolding stroke slowly along the top and bottom of their foot until your fingertips slide off the tips of their toes. Repeat a couple of times.

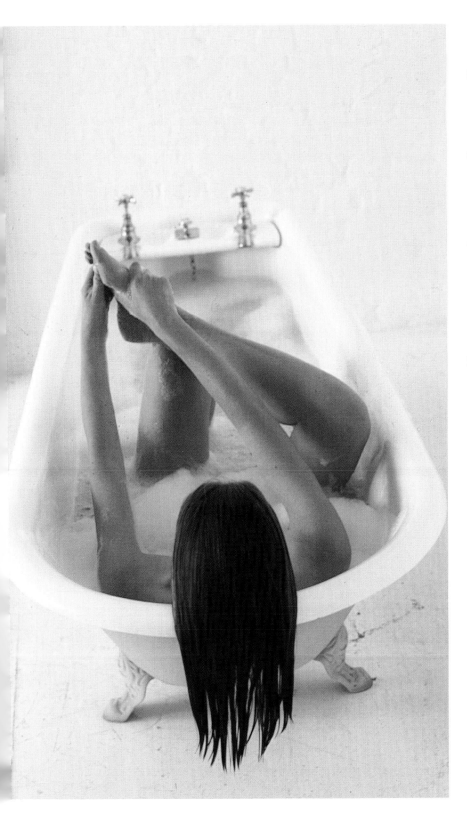

diy massage

● **feet**

1 **Place one foot across the opposite knee and massage the whole sole using both your thumbs in firm, rotating movements** (left)**. Finish by squeezing and pulling each toe.**

troubleshooters

Warm and stimulate cold feet by massaging with two or three drops of rosemary essence in a carrier oil. Or add a pinch of mustard to a bowl of hot water and soak the feet for ten minutes.

●

Find the solar plexus area on your sole – it is approximately 5cm (2in) below the middle toe. It is said that by pressing and stimulating this area you will energize your sensual feelings!

●

An easy and efficient way of giving yourself a foot massage is to use a massage tool designed for the job. Or, just grab a rolling pin and use that instead. Place it on the floor, put your bare foot on top of it and move your foot backwards and forwards, moving the rolling pin back and forth under your sole.

●

Ease aching feet by rubbing them with lemon juice. Also, soaking feet in warm water that has had a few drops of peppermint oil added to it, is bliss!

aromatherapy

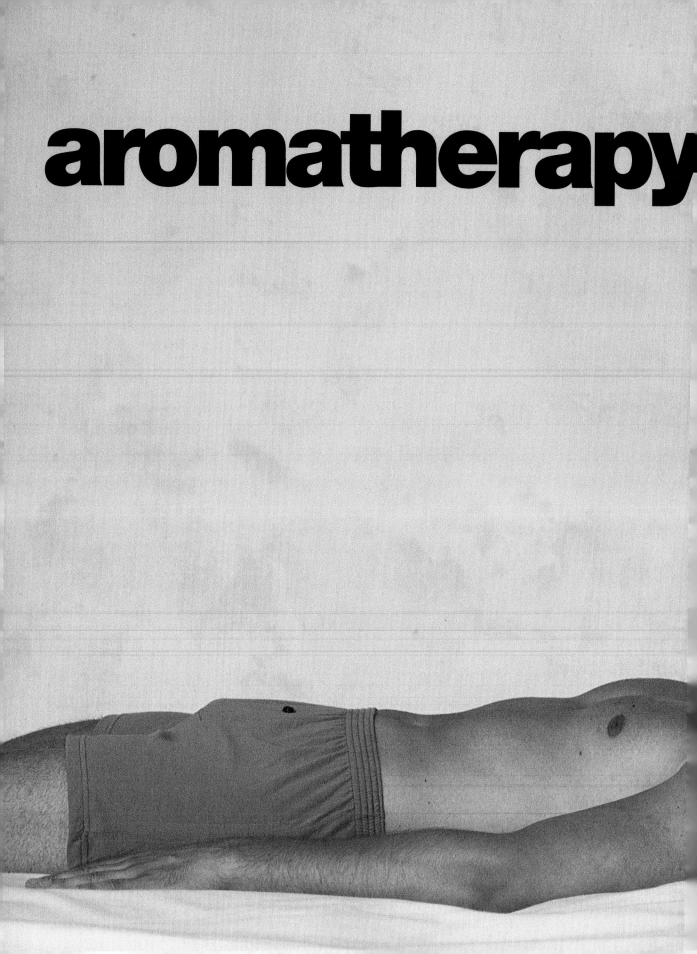

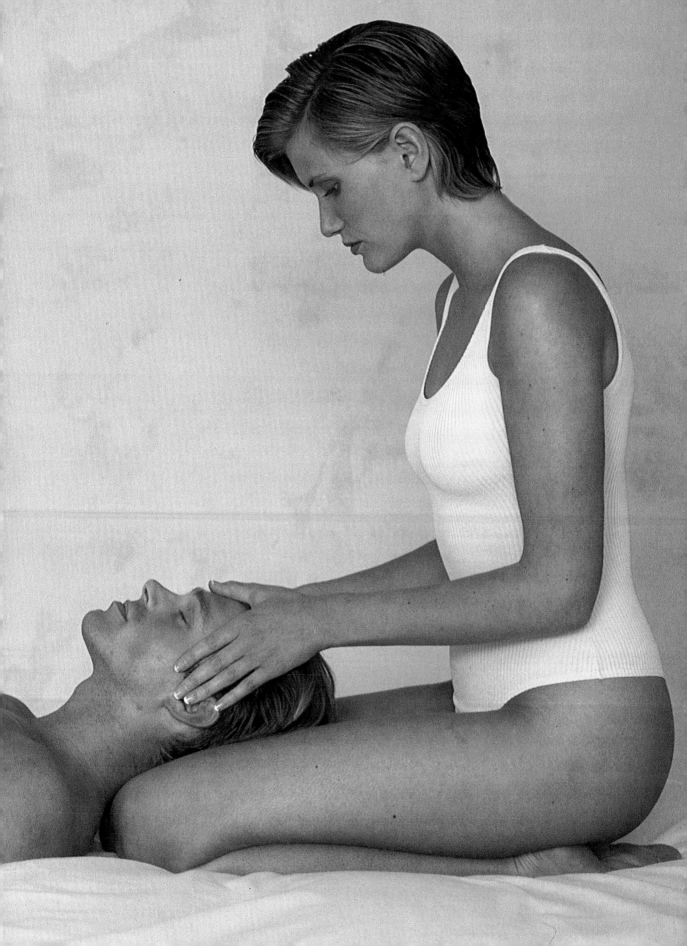

although not a specific massage technique in itself, aromatherapy is synonymous with relaxation.

In aromatherapy, essential oils – the aromatic extracts taken from flowers, plants and herbs – are used to treat a wide variety of ailments, both physical and emotional. Although it has only become popular again within the last ten years, aromatherapy has been around for about 3,000 years.

According to practitioners, every essential oil has a unique healing property and works not only on our physical body, but on our psyche too. The medium in which essential oils are used can vary from inhalation, where oils are vaporized in boiling water, to topical application through massage. The latter has been found to be one of the most effective methods, as it combines the power of touch with that of smell, triggering a complex chain of reactions within the brain. The inhalation of essential oils stimulates the olfactory receptors that pass messages to the limbic system, the part of the brain in which feelings and emotions are processed and controlled.

In aromatherapy massage, essential oils are mixed with a carrier oil and applied to the skin. Aromatherapists maintain that essential oils, unlike most other substances, can penetrate the skin, whereupon they are absorbed into the bloodstream. Essential oils should be used externally only. They can be highly toxic if used incorrectly and should never be used neat, as they are highly concentrated substances.

Most aromatherapists use lymphatic drainage techniques, acupressure points and Swedish massage strokes, but they also use special movements developed by the French biochemist and grandmother of aromatherapy, Marguerite Maury. One of the things a therapist will focus on is the body's energy channels, or meridians, which were originally discovered and worked on by ancient Chinese practitioners. The aim of an aromatherapy massage is to release muscle tension and thereby allow energy to flow freely throughout the body. In turn, this helps stimulate the smooth functioning of vital organs, nerves, glands, blood circulation and the lymphatic system – the body's 'waste disposal' network. The result can be either relaxing or invigorating, depending on the oil chosen and its particular properties.

In France, many doctors train to be aromatherapists, believing that essential oils have potent healing powers. Research at the University of Montpelier's Faculty of Aromatherapy has backed up many of the traditional claims that have been made about aromatherapy, such as the ability of certain oils to trigger a relaxation response. In Japan, scientists at the University of Tokyo have also found that essential oils work on the nervous system to affect the physiology of both mind and body.

While you need to be a qualified aromatherapist to treat serious medical problems, everyone can use aromatherapy to enhance the effect of massage. For example, if you want to relax the person you are massaging, or if you are practising self-massage, lavender, vetiver and ylang ylang all have soothing and calming properties. Alternatively, you can uplift spirits by using rosemary.

blending essential oils

As essential oils should be used diluted, you need a 'carrier oil' to transport them to your skin. There are plenty of vegetable, nut and seed oils you can use as carrier oils. See pages 19–21 for some suggestions.

When mixing essential oils with a carrier oil, a rough guide is to use one drop of essential oil to 2 ml (½ tsp) of carrier oil. So, 50 ml (1⅔ fl oz) of carrier oil, which is roughly what you'd use for a full body massage, can contain up to 25 drops of essential oils. For a facial oil, the dilution ratio changes. For normal skin, two to three drops of essential oil to every 10 ml (⅓ fl oz) of carrier oil is a reasonable mix. If skin is super sensitive, use a less concentrated blend of oils; try just one drop per 10 ml (⅓ fl oz).

Choose your essential oils for their physical and emotional therapeutic benefits. Ask the person you're massaging if they feel they have any specific problems which need particular attention. It's important that they actually like the aroma of the massage oil so let them smell your blend and make comments on it before you start.

guide to essential oils

basil

physical uses: anti-depressant, antiseptic, good for digestive problems, headaches, sinusitis, colds, asthma.
emotional uses: nervous tension, anxiety, stress.
contraindications/comments: avoid if pregnant; dilute well to protect against possible skin irritation; good insect repellent.

benzoin

physical uses: healing, diuretic, aids circulation, antiseptic, good for asthma, arthritis, cystitis, cracked, sore and irritated skin.
emotional uses: anxiety, unhappiness.
contraindications/comments: benzoin has been known to cause allergic skin reactions. If you often suffer skin irritation, it's wise to do a patch test with this oil. Simply apply a drop, on a cotton bud, to the crook of your elbow. Leave it for 24 hours, then check for redness or irritation. If there's no reaction you can use it safely.

bergamot

physical uses: anti-depressant, analgesic, good for skincare, including problems such as acne and eczema, relieves urinary infections.
emotional uses: uplifting.
contraindications/comments: avoid if sunbathing, as it makes the skin photosensitive.

camomile

physical uses: digestive problems, fevers, PMT, toothache, migraine, irritability, dermatitis, antiseptic.
emotional uses: calming, soothing, restores equilibrium.
contraindications/comment: can be used very effectively and safely for children.

clary sage

physical uses: sedative, astringent, aphrodisiac, antiseptic, helpful for PMT and as a tonic for the reproductive organs.
emotional uses: stress, exhaustion.
contraindications/comments: avoid if pregnant; it can produce a mild form of euphoric intoxication, but beware, large doses will produce a headache.

cypress

physical uses: diuretic, astringent, antiseptic, soothes influenza and coughs, useful for menopausal problems, varicose and broken veins, cellulite, PMT.
emotional uses: nervous tension

eucalyptus

physical uses: analgesic, antiseptic, expectorant, relieves fevers, coughs, cystitis, migraine, diabetes, muscular pains, all respiratory disorders.
contraindications/comments: good insect repellent.

fennel

physical uses: cleansing, aids all digestive problems, cellulite, kidney stones, fluid retention, eases urinary problems.
Contraindications/comments: avoid during pregnancy; during breastfeeding however, fennel aids milk production when supply is low.

geranium

physical uses: anti-depressant, mildly diuretic, eases PMT and menopausal symptoms, normalizes all skin types.
emotional uses: uplifting, balancing.

juniper

physical uses: cleansing, diuretic, purifying, antiseptic, helps cystitis, painful periods, acne, cellulite, fluid retention, aching joints.

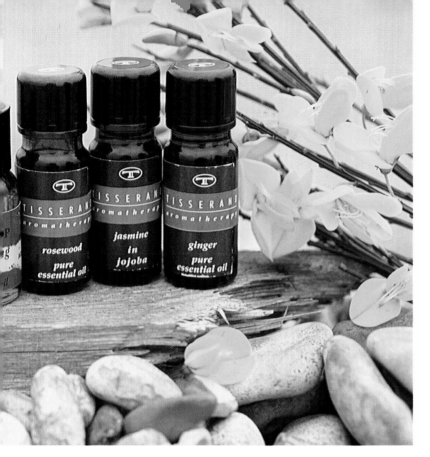

tive skin.
emotional uses: can help frigidi-ty/impotence, uplifting.

sandalwood
physical uses: diuretic, tonic, anti-depressant, antiseptic, aphrodisiac, relives cystitis, acne, coughs, fluid retention.
emotional uses: uplifting, soothes anxiety, used by some to treat frigidity/impotence.
contraindications/comment: although today felling of sandal-wood trees is strictly controlled, large scale destruction in the past and illegal cutting have meant that in some areas the tree's future is unsure. Replanting programmes are in operation, but it you'd like to substitute sandalwood for another oil, try galbanum, whose properties are not dissimilar.

tangerine
physical uses: tonic, aids insom-nia, stomach pains.
emotional uses: anxiety, uplift-ing, revitalizing.
contraindications/comments: good to use during pregnancy and on children.

tea tree
physical uses: antiseptic, anti-fungal, treats thrush, cystitis, candida, respiratory infections, colds, acne, rashes.
contraindications/comments: can be used undiluted on spots, cold sores, bites etc.

ylang ylang
physical uses: aphrodisiac, anti-depressant, high blood pres-sure, insomnia, tension, oily skin.
emotional uses: calming, can help frigidity/impotence.
contraindications/comments: has a strong, sweet smell, but beware, too much can make you feel nauseous or give you a headache.

contraindications/comments: some aromatherapists suggest avoiding juniper during pregnancy.

lavender
physical uses: anti-depressant, antiseptic, analgesic, good for all skin care, respiratory infec-tions, insomnia, fever, digestive problems, menstrual problems.
emotional uses: manic depres-sion, nervous exhaustion.
contraindications/comments: a multi-purpose oil, which can also be used neat – on spots, stings or burns for example.

lemongrass
physical uses: antiseptic, colitis, wind, fluid retention, acne
contraindications /comments: good insect repellent. Take care when using on very sensitive skin.

marjoram
physical uses: pain-relieving, sedative, aphrodisiac, helps PMT, sprained joints, insomnia,

colds, asthma, high blood pres-sure, constipation.
emotional uses: anxiety, calming.
contraindication/comments: avoid if pregnant.

neroli (orange blossom)
physical uses: aphrodisiac, anti-depressant, antiseptic, helps stress-induced stomach disor-ders, sensitive/irritated skin, poor circulation.
emotional uses: unhappiness, de-stresser, shock.

peppermint
physical uses: stimulating, tonic, analgesic, antiseptic, astringent, fights diarrhoea, headache, colds, asthma, bronchitis, nau-sea, muscular pain, general fatigue, neuralgia, sunburn.

rose
physical uses: anti-depressant, aphrodisiac, antiseptic, tonic, eases headaches, nerves, helps irregular periods, all skin types, but especially dry/older/sensi-

special massage blends

● **acne, treatment** 10 ml (⅓ fl oz) grapeseed or sweet almond oil, 5 drops juniper oil – apply a couple of times a day to the affected area during flare-ups.

● **anxiety/depression soother** 10 ml (⅓ fl oz) carrier oil, 3 drops neroli – rub onto solar plexus, back of the neck and in circular movements around the temples. Sit quietly and relax for a few minutes.

● **athlete's foot remedy** 15 ml (½ fl oz) carrier oil, 10 drops geranium oil – massage into the feet morning and evening.

● **insomnia blend** (for use when accompanied by nervous fatigue) 15 ml (½ fl oz) carrier oil, 4 drops nutmeg, 3 drops rosemary, 8 drops marjoram – use as a relaxing massage oil before bed.

● **varicose vein reliever** 50 ml (1⅔ fl oz) carrier oil, 15 drops cypress – lightly massage into the legs each day.

looking after your essential oils

Essential oils are volatile and sensitive. They can evaporate quickly and are easily damaged by being exposed to sunlight and heat. To help them stay in peak condition, keep them in very dark glass bottles (i.e. amber/brown or blue) or metal containers with airtight lids. Store them in a cool, dark place.

● **end of the day massage oil** 50 ml (1⅔ fl oz) carrier oil, 10 drops geranium, 10 drops lavender, 5 drops marjoram – use as an all-over relaxing body massage oil.

● **pregnancy stretchmark prevention** 10 ml (⅓ fl oz) carrier oil, to include 2 ml (½ tsp) wheatgerm oil with 4 drops of either of the following, singly or in combination – lavender, tangerine and neroli. Massage into the abdomen, hips, tops of thighs and bottom every day.

● **circulation booster** 50 ml (1⅔ fl oz) carrier oil, 10 drops neroli, 10 drops rose and 5 drops cypress. A total body tonic that helps to stimulate a sluggish circulation.

● **tired leg remedy** 10 ml (⅓ fl oz) carrier oil, 4 to 5 drops of clary sage. Massage from ankles to just above the knees. Then sit with your feet higher than your head for 10 to 15 minutes.

● **headache soother** 5 ml (1 tsp) carrier oil, with 1 or 2 drops of either basil, lavender, camomile, clary sage or juniper. Massage the blend into the back of the neck, the base of the head, temples, forehead and around the eyes.

aromatherapy body massage

An aromatherapy massage is mainly based on intuition – if it feels good, keep doing it! Here are some moves we guarantee will feel wonderful. You can incorporate movements from the other chapters in his book too or just invent your own. We begin with the massage recipient lying on their stomach.

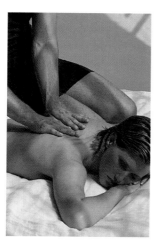

1 **Warm the aromatherapy oil in your hands then stroke it onto the back. With your hands flat either side of the spine, slowly but firmly work up the back from the base in one long stroking movement** (above). **When you reach the neck, move your hands out over the shoulders and down the top of the arms. Glide your hands back to the base of the spine, using little or no pressure. Repeat a few times.**

2 **Kneel at the side of your partner, hands flat and at one side in the centre of their back** (right). **Rest the tips of your fingers on the ridge at the side of their spine. Slowly slide one hand up along the side of the back towards their shoulders. The other hand slides down towards their buttocks. Bring your hands gently back to the central starting position and repeat the same movements three or four times. Then repeat on the other side of the back.**

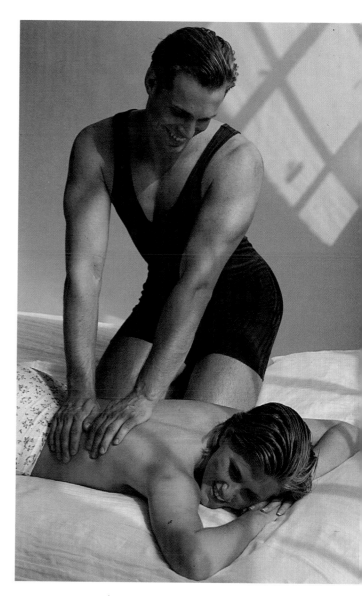

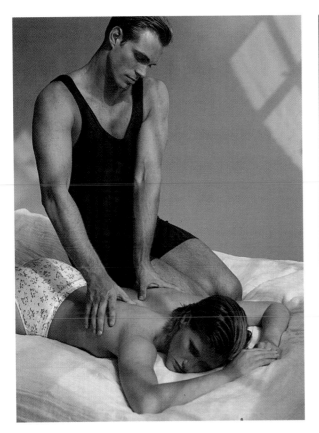

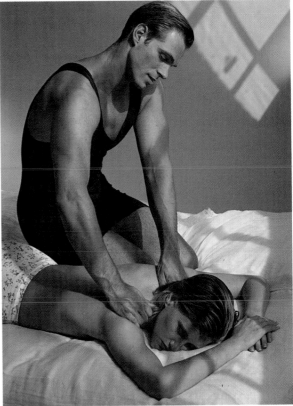

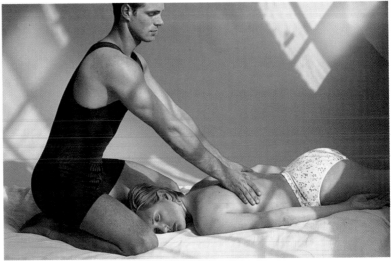

3 In the same kneeling position, turn so you face up your partner's body, towards their head (above left). With your hands at the bottom of their back, place your thumbs either side of their spine. Work up the back using small up and out movements with your thumbs. Finish at the base of your partner's neck.

4 Now massage the shoulders with a kneading action, helping to relieve any knots and tension you may find there (above right).

5 Sit above your partner's head and work down either side of the spine using your thumbs, i.e. step 3 in reverse (above).

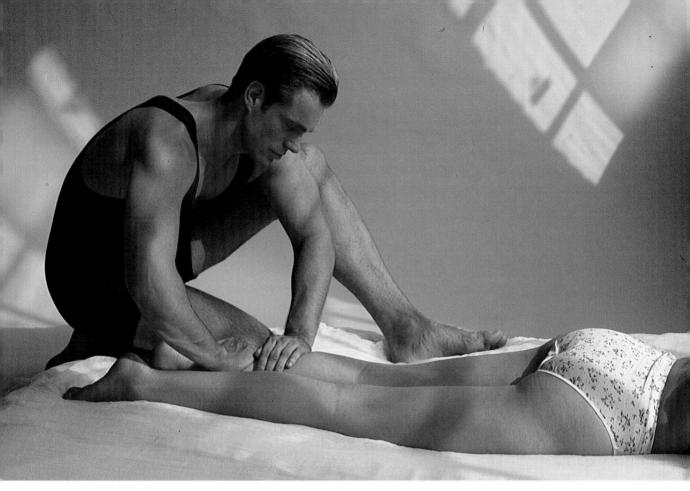

6 Without losing contact with your partner's body, move to the side of their lower legs (left or right) and stroke firmly upwards from their ankles towards their buttocks. Trail your hands back down and repeat (above).

7 From the same position, use kneading movements over both their calves and over the backs of their thighs.

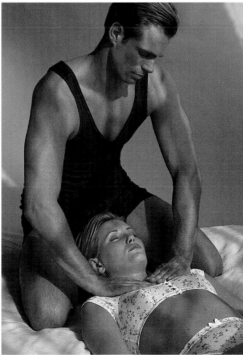

8 Ask your partner to turn over, then repeat the firm stroking movement, working from the ankles to the tops of the thighs.

9 Now return to the position above your partner's head and massage from the centre of their chest out over the shoulders and down their upper arms (left).

aromatherapy facial massage

A facial massage using essential oils not only feels wonderful, but will improve your complexion too, as it stimulates the micro-circulation. The result is an instantly glowing, healthier-looking skin. Performed on a regular basis, facial massage ensures clear, blooming skin. Some people say it's almost as good as a facelift. It's easily incorporated into your skincare routine – you can do most of the following moves on yourself, though it is great to be pampered sometimes by having someone else give you the massage. You can use the moves below by themselves or in a combination with the strokes described in the full massage sequence on pages 85-87.

1 **Lightly stroke your chosen aromatherapy blend over the face and neck. Use simple, sweeping, up and out movements** (right)**.**

2 **Working from the centre of the chin to the ears, pinch along the jaw-bone using your thumbs and forefingers. Pinch, release, then slide your fingers along half a centimetre (a quarter of an inch) before pinching again.**

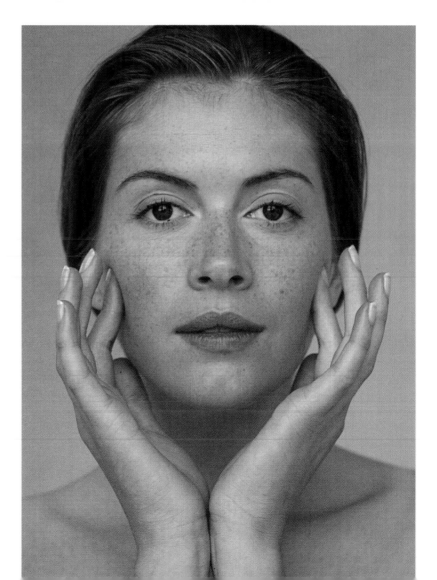

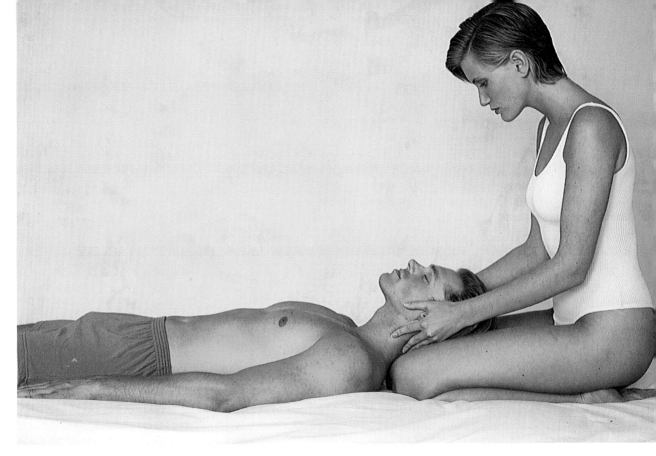

● **If you're massaging someone else, you should be behind their head.**

3 Place your thumbs together under your chin and your forefingers by your nostrils. Press with your fingers, then release and continue this movement, working down the lines that run from the nose to the corner of the mouth. Repeat without removing your supporting fingers.

4 Using your forefingers (or thumbs) stroke from the inner corners of your eyes and down the sides of your nose. Repeat several times.

5 Using the same pinching and releasing movements as in step 2, work from the inner corner of the eyebrows to the outer corners.

6 Now use all your fingers to press along the underside of your cheekbones, working all the way out to your ears. Repeat as often as you wish, then stroke the same area in a sweeping movement.

7 With alternate hands, stroke your fingers up and out over your forehead. Perform this stroke over both cheeks and up the neck.

8 Lightly tap your fingers all over the face, then rest your hand on the forehead and over the eyes for a few seconds to finish the treatment.

part 2

sensua
massac
reflex

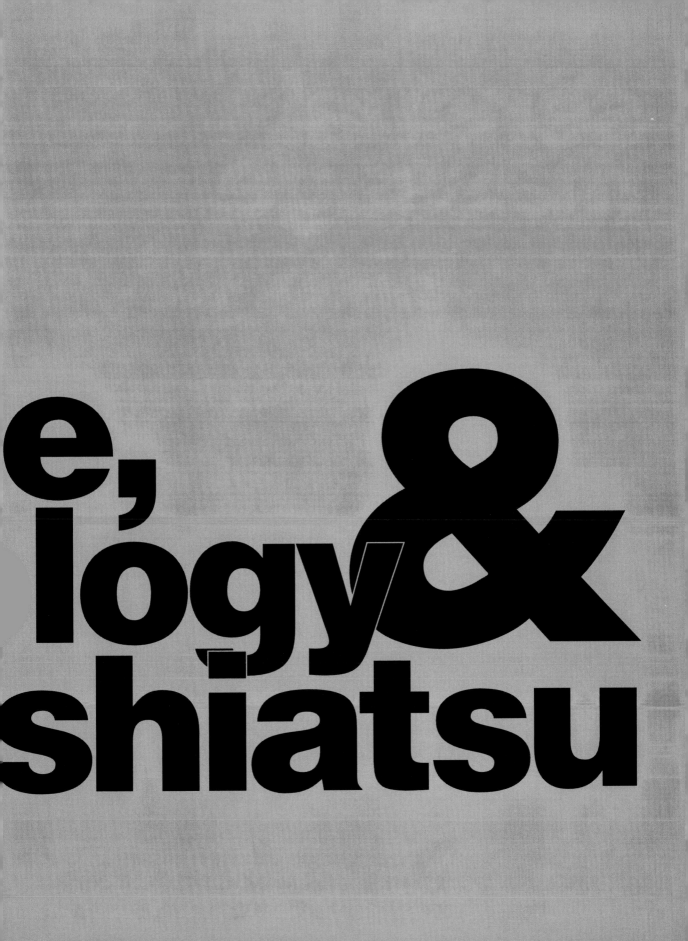

sensual
massage

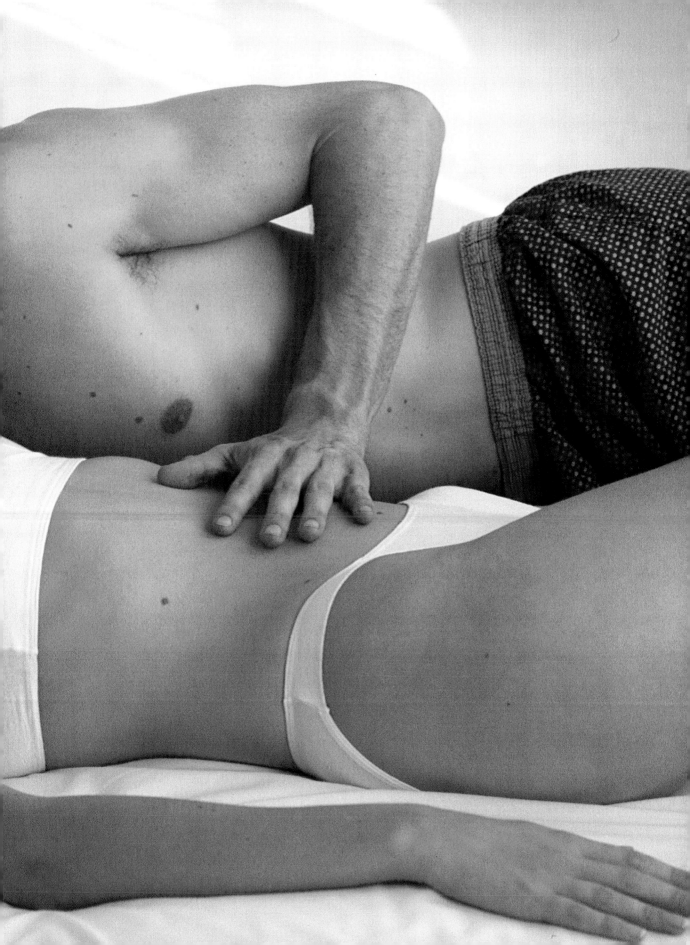

to the uninitiated in Western cultures, the word massage is full of innuendo, having been given, mistakenly, a sexual connotation. Many people, especially men, are apprehensive about going for a professional massage for this very reason, fearing that they will find it sexually stimulating. Although a massage invariably feels wonderful whether from the hands of a trained practitioner or an amateur, it rarely feels sexual. For a massage to feel truly sensual, and sexual in any way, there have to be existing loving feelings between both partners.

In the context of a long-term relationship, massage is a potent therapy. The feelings of closeness, security and sincerity it engenders means that you can maintain, enhance, even mend, a relationship on a physical, emotional and spiritual level. Regular massage sessions together could help you stay partners for life. Try it – we promise you won't be disappointed.

You'll find that sensual massage works in a number of ways. It can be more pleasurable than intercourse – the discovery of new ways to make your partner feel good can be deeply satisfying for both of you. And afterwards, imagine the bliss of simply curling up together and falling asleep in each other's arms. Massage can also be used as sexual foreplay through exploration. Sometimes you can't help but focus on the obvious erogenous zones such as buttocks, breasts and genitals, but you can also find new, surprisingly sensitive areas of your partner's body that may well increase their desire and pleasure. Naturally everyone likes different things, but as a starting point, try massaging your partner's feet, the backs of their knees, the crooks of the elbows and around their ears.

As you massage, feel the texture of your partner's skin. Feel the muscles, bones, curves and angles. Vary the strokes you use and the pressure you apply. A softer touch will be most sexually stimulating. Gentle tickling is good too, helping to break down any inhibitions! Above all, remember that sensual massage with your partner is for enjoyment. We have suggested some initial moves, but the best will undoubtedly be your own.

● **when not to massage** Don't start your sensual massage if you're going to be interrupted. This is time for just the two of you and your relationship. Treat it as a special occasion and it will be so. Don't attempt to massage your partner if you feel very tired, as you should put effort into it – it won't feel convincing if you don't. And, if your partner is very tired, don't massage them – you'll be cross if they fall asleep!

sensual essentials

Use your touch in combination with essential oils to enhance the sensual experience. The following are the sexiest of oils to add to a carrier oil: ylang-ylang, rose, sandalwood, rosemary, jasmine and neroli.

● **getting in the mood** For sensual massage, the main ingredient is privacy. This is one time when you really don't want to be disturbed, so lock the door and take the phone off the hook – whatever it takes to make sure that the time you set aside is just for the two of you.

The massage surface you use is

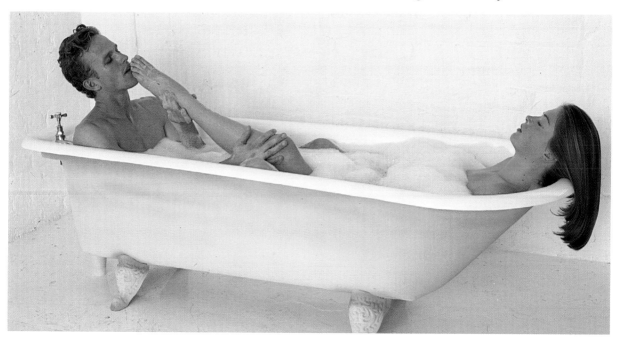

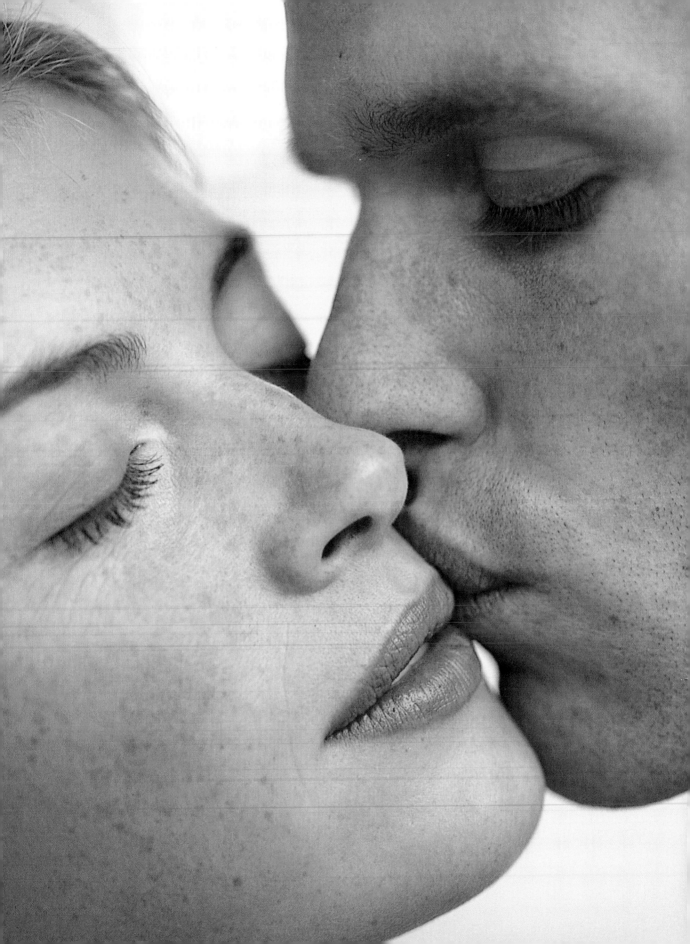

up to you, but it should be comfortable and reasonably firm. You could set up a 'bed' next to the fire for example, using plenty of cushions and blankets.

Whatever time of day you choose for your massage, you should try to ensure the pace is unhurried. A Sunday morning is ideal, midweek before going to work is probably not! A sensuality-filled evening is perhaps the most obvious choice. While spontaneity is wonderful, if you plan a special evening with your partner, the day-long anticipation that leads up to it can be quite a turn-on in itself. Ring each other at lunchtime and tell your partner that you love them and that you can't wait to get home. When you do get home, relax together first in a warm bath or shower and get the day's problems and news over with. Put on your favourite music, light candles or burn essential oils. Have a drink, a special meal… enjoy.

taoist sensual massage

For those interested in taking sensual massage a little further, we recommend some further reading on Taoism, the ancient Chinese healing philosophy. In Taoism, massage is used to encourage the free flow of *Chi*, or life force, around the body. Specific organs are stimulated for total physical and mental well being. When energy flows freely via the energy channels, or meridians, pleasure is experienced and this sets up a chain reaction. For instance, massaging your earlobes will not only mean that you get a warm feeling in them, but you may also feel a tingling sensation in your lower back.

Ching Chi, or sexual energy, is, according to Taoist belief, the most basic in our bodies. A Taoist doctor can actually prescribe sexual techniques too as a form of healing, just as a Western doctor would probably give drugs. In combination with other methods of healing, such as acupuncture, the Taoist method of healing the body certainly makes the road to recovery lots of fun.

In the sequence that follows, we have included some Taoist moves as well as other sensual techniques. But remember, it's you and your partner that matter, so just do what feels right at the time.

sensual massage sequence

1 Using a small amount of massage oil, undiluted or with essential oils added, gently stroke your partner's feet. Work from the toes up over the feet towards the ankles and up to the calves. Stroke, press, rub and even kiss the toes and soles of the feet (right). **Try to spend at least a few minutes on each foot.**

2 Ask your partner to lie on their back if they are not already doing so. Separate their legs and kneel in between them, facing upwards towards their head. The Taoist movement you are about to perform is called Flying on the Land – because if you were to walk afterwards, you would feel as if you were floating. It is intended to give your partner feelings of safety and security, as well as stabilizing their sexual energy. Push your palms up the inside of the shinbones, up and over the knees and down on the other side of the shinbone. Move from the outer ankle to the inner ankle and back up the inside of the shinbone again. Repeat this movement for about a minute, asking your partner to breathe with you as you do it – inhaling when your hands work up and exhaling as they move back down. Make your touch lighter with each repetition.

3 Now work on your partner's thighs. With both hands at the knees, work your palms up the inner thighs. Run your fingers across the dip where the thighs meet the body, over and outwards. Pull your palms down the outside of the thighs as far as the knees and repeat.

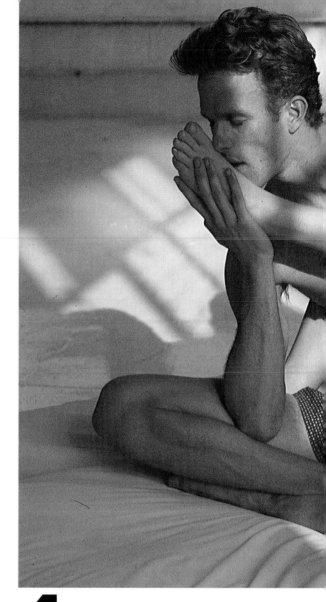

4 Move to one side of your partner's upper body. Place one hand below and the other above your partner's navel, then move them together in a clockwise circle (right). As you repeat the movement make your touch softer. Digestive problems, cramps and anxiety will be soothed with this movement. Equally, the Taoists say that it stimulates sexual energy stored in the pelvic region.

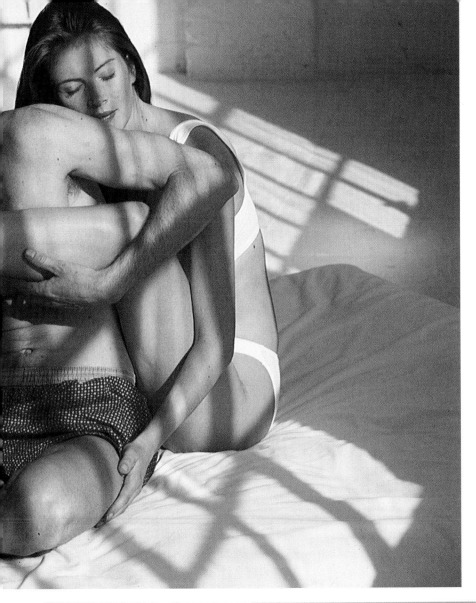

5 Stroke your hands over your partner's chest, out over their shoulders and down their arms to their hands.

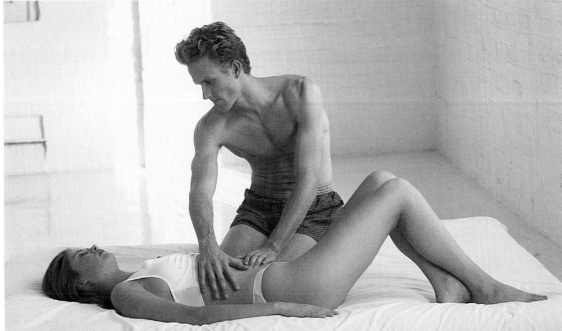

99

6 Now concentrate on one arm at a time. Take your partner's hand and turn it gently so that it's palm up (top right). Using your flattened fingertips, press along the mid-line of the arm from the palm to the elbow, pausing slightly, then move on to the upper arms (right). Run your fingers over your partner's shoulder, then down the mid-line of the outside of the arm to the hand. Repeat slowly using a gentle touch for a minute or so on each arm.

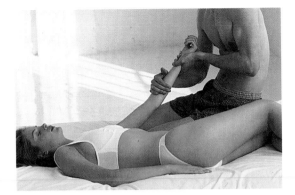

7 Ask your partner to sit up slowly. Before getting them to lie on their stomach, spend a few minutes gently kneading and stroking their shoulders and neck (below). A few kisses are highly recommended at this point too! You could also try massaging your partner's head – just as though you were gently shampooing their hair.

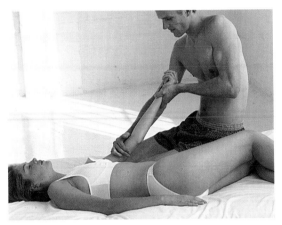

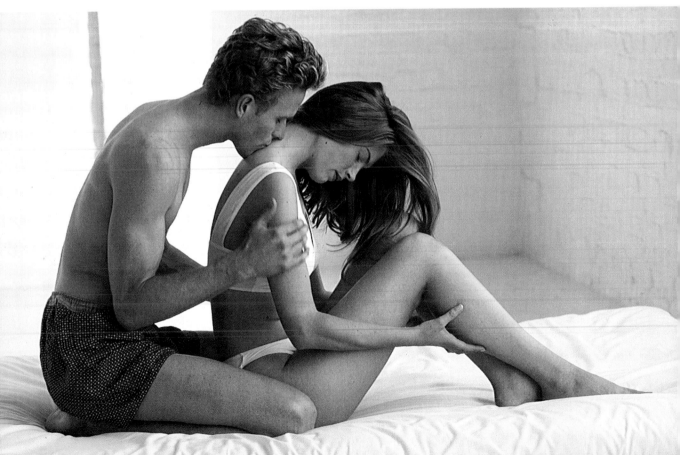

8

Now ask your partner to lie on their stomach. The next move helps to release the spine and muscles that surround it. As you perform the stroke, imagine that you are lengthening the spine and clearing away tension. Begin by kneeling behind your partner between their legs and place your left hand on their lower back and let it 'settle' into the sacrum. Put your right hand, palm flat, fingers pointing towards your partner's head, in front of your left hand along the spine. With your hand flat, slowly push your right palm up the spine until you reach the base of the skull. The stroke should take around 20 seconds. Repeat for three minutes or so, gently increasing the pressure of your right hand, but keeping your left hand steady. This move is the Taoist Climbing the Column, which should leave your partner feeling wonderfully energized.

9

Move to kneel in front of your partner's head. The following move will 'lengthen' the spine further, release tension, soothe muscle aches and make your partner feel 'lighter' (below). With your hands either side of the spine, palms flat, fingers pointing down your partner's body, push your hands down their back. Use your body weight for pressure.

When you reach the sacrum, push your palms out sideways to the hips, then move them up the sides of your partner's body to their armpits. Circle their shoulders, then you'll be back in the starting position. Repeat for a few minutes, then press and rotate your thumbs either side of the spine, working downwards. Finish by stroking your fingers lightly up to the shoulders.

10

Move down again to kneel between your partner's legs. Starting at the inner ankle, lightly stroke up the inner calves and thighs. Then separate your hands over your partner's buttocks and move them out to the hips. From there, pull your hands down over the outer thighs and calves, with your thumbs tracing a line in the middle of the legs. Repeat slowly for a few minutes.

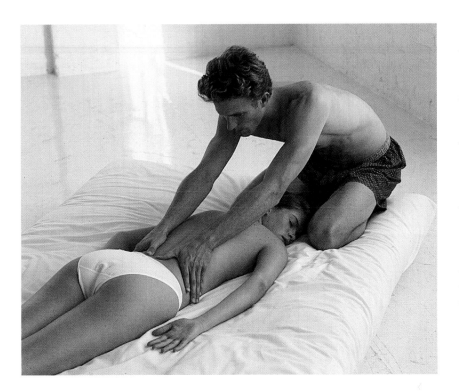

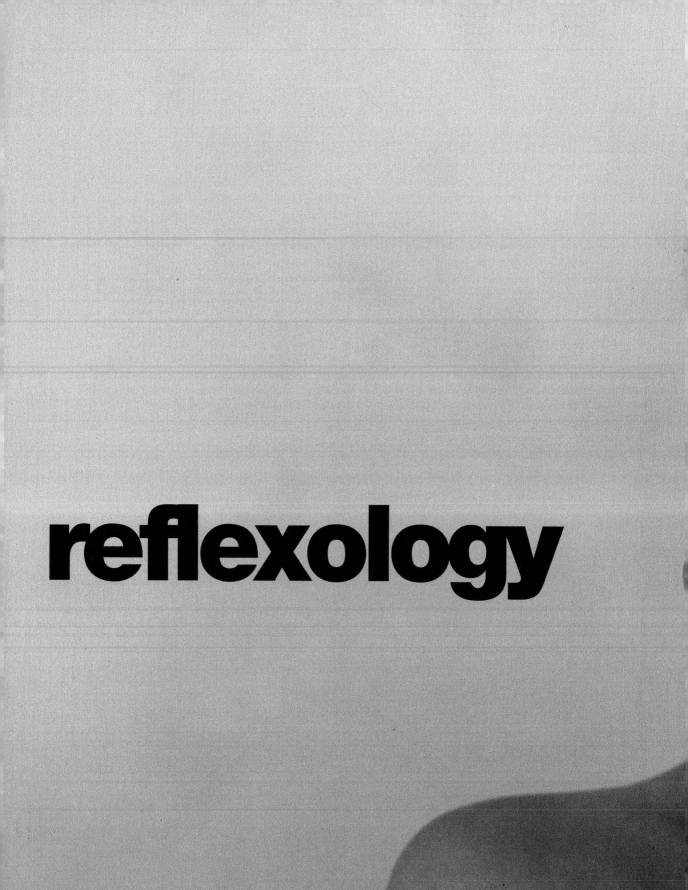

reflexology

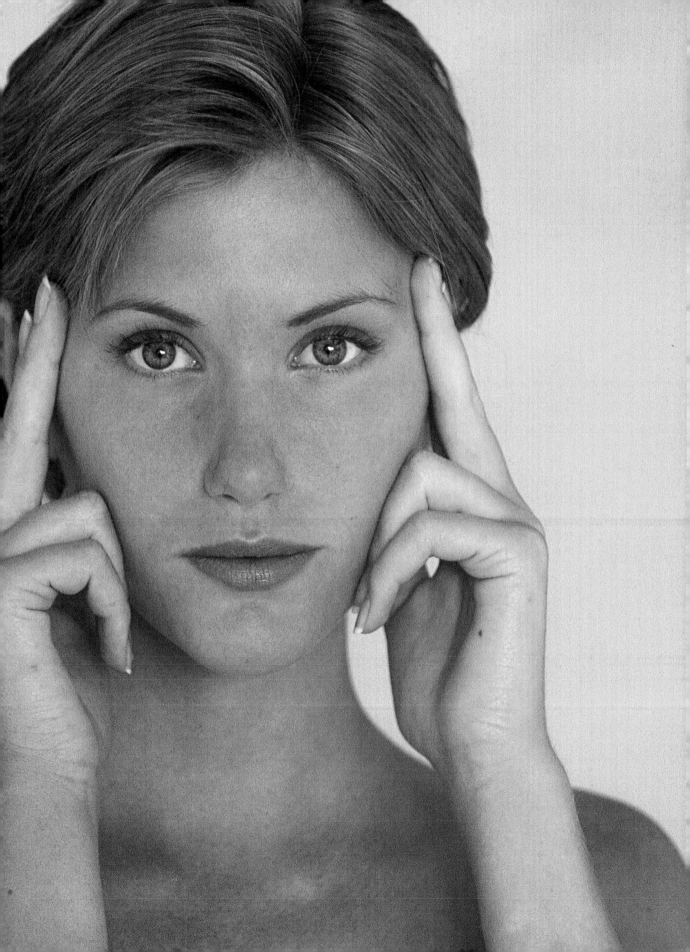

for some, a hand and foot massage is the ultimate pleasure. There is also no doubt that it's beneficial to both our physical and our emotional well being.

Used by Chinese practitioners to treat and diagnose illness, the massage and manipulation of the hands and feet, known as reflexology, has been used in the East for thousands of years. While not strictly a massage technique in its own right, the basis for this treatment is to stimulate pressure points on the hands and feet using a variety of strokes.

In the early 1900s, an American doctor named William Fitzgerald was investigating the link between the hands and feet and the rest of the body. Fitzgerald's work suggested that there are ten zones, or energy channels, running vertically through the body – five on either side. All of these zones are connected to the hands and feet and linked to the body's major organs. He believed that by pressing points on the hands and feet, specific organs in the body were directly affected.

Eunice Ingham, a physiotherapist and masseuse, reinforced Fitzgerald's theory in the 1930s by 'mapping' the areas on the hands and feet that correspond to the rest of the body. This enabled reflexology practitioners to determine accurately which area to press in order to treat specific problems. It is also believed that when certain areas on the feet are tender or lumpy, the related organ within that zone may need treatment. For example, by pressing the centre of the right foot, you can stimulate the liver which is in the corresponding zone. The lumpy areas are supposedly crystalline deposits of uric acid and calcium that form at the nerve endings and prevent it from functioning at optimum efficiency. When pressure is applied to these deposits, they are broken down, reabsorbed by the bloodstream and excreted in the urine. In addition, by pressing on the nerve endings, the entire nerve is stimulated and as a result, a complex chain of reactions is triggered in that particular zone. In essence, the hands and the feet can be used by a therapist to communicate with the whole body. Although it would be unwise to use reflexology for self-diagnosis, you can use it to promote relaxation and relieve stress.

Before performing any reflexology, examine the charts below and on page 106 which detail the areas of the hands and feet which correspond to the major organs of the body. *Note:* Do not perform reflexology on anyone less than 12 weeks pregnant.

reflexology preparation

You don't need to remove all of your clothes for reflexology. Just ask the recipient to take off their shoes and socks/tights, and any jewellery, and you can begin.

Before you start the treatment, the recipient should relax by soaking their feet in warm water for a few minutes. This softens calloused skin, stimulates the blood flow and can help make the treatment more effective.

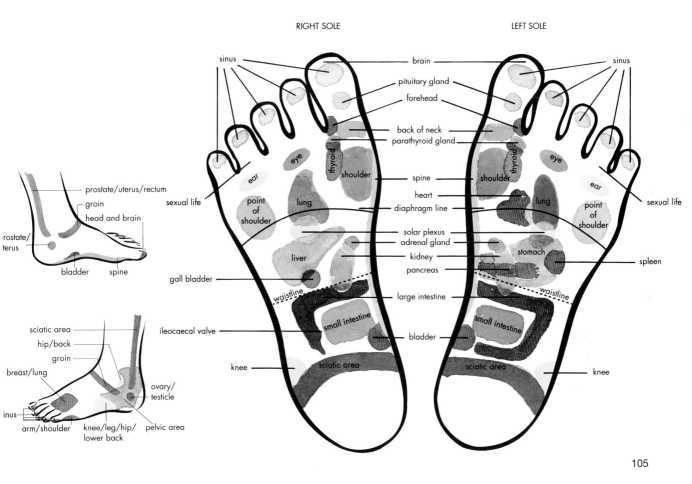

reflexology

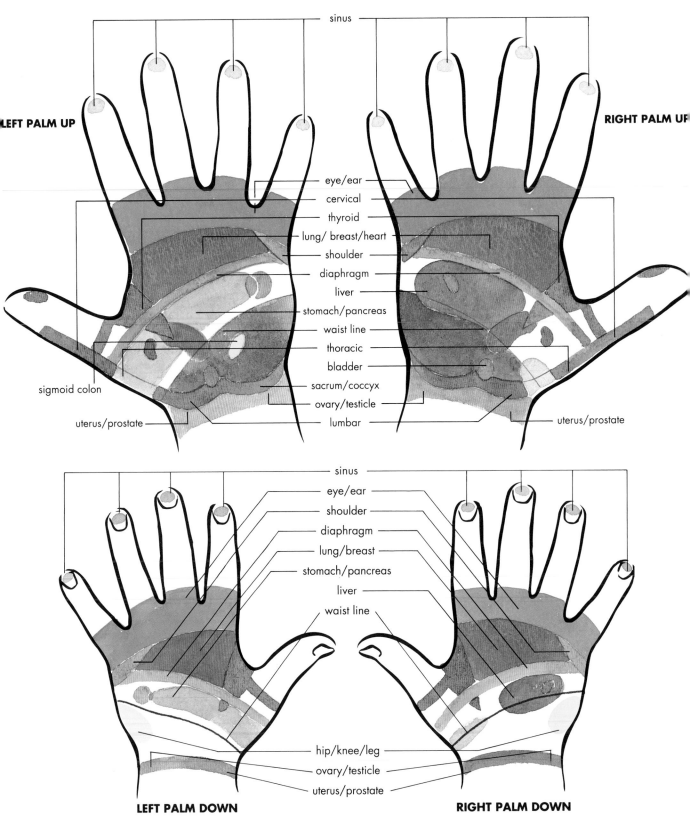

sinus

LEFT PALM UP
RIGHT PALM UP

eye/ear
cervical
thyroid
lung/ breast/heart
shoulder
diaphragm
liver
stomach/pancreas
waist line
thoracic
bladder
sacrum/coccyx
ovary/testicle
lumbar

sigmoid colon

uterus/prostate

uterus/prostate

sinus
eye/ear
shoulder
diaphragm
lung/breast
stomach/pancreas
liver
waist line

hip/knee/leg
ovary/testicle
uterus/prostate

LEFT PALM DOWN
RIGHT PALM DOWN

When practising a reflexology sequence you can sit on the floor or on a bed at your partner's feet. Ensure that your partner is propped up with pillows to support their back, and place a few cushions under their knees and lower legs so that you can have easy access to all the areas of the feet and ankles. Or you might find it easier to sit with their feet rested on your knees. You shouldn't use oil when performing reflexology – a little talcum powder works best. Work gently and steadily. Your partner may experience discomfort. This could signify that there is a problem in the organ connected to the zone you are working on so, unless it's very painful, spend a few moments concentrating on that spot.

basic strokes

There are a wide variety of strokes which are used in reflexology. Below are six of the main moves used on the hands and feet:

● **thumb walking** Bend the outer edge of the thumb at the first joint and move it along the foot in small steps. You can practise by pressing the outer edge of your thumb on a smooth surface, such as a table. Bend it and slide it along repeatedly, using the tiniest movements possible while maintaining a consistent pressure (*overleaf, above right*).

● **finger walking** Use the corner edge of the index finger to take small steps along the hands or feet. If you are working down a long area, such as the side of the foot, use two fingers in tandem (*overleaf, above left*).

● **rotation on a point** Use this movement when you are working on points that may be tender. If you are using thumb pressure on one of the adrenal glands for example, you can gently hold the toes with the other hand and rotate them gently (*overleaf, below*).

● **pivot on a point** This is an alternative to the rotation move. While you are using one thumb to keep pressure on the point, use your other hand to press the foot back and away from you, and onto your thumb. Hold the foot firmly with your hand, letting your fingers rest across the top of the foot, over the ankle. As your thumb walks diagonally across the reflex, twist the foot away from you and then back again in a gentle and rhythmical

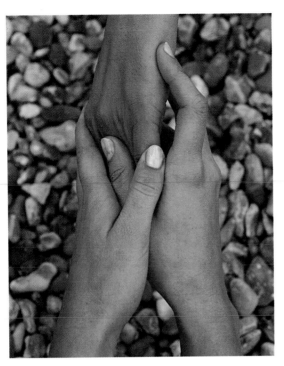

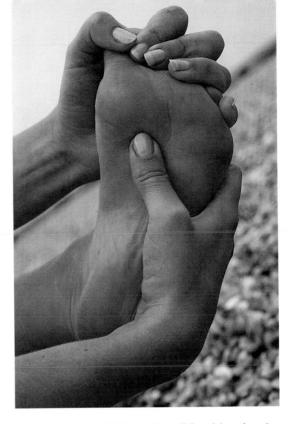

● **Basic techniques: finger walking** (above left), **thumb walking** (above), **rotation on a point** (left).

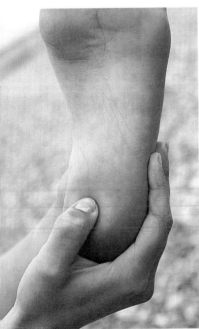

movement. It sounds more complicated than it is. Once you have tried it a few times, it will become second nature.

● **flexing on a point** This is similar to the previous move but instead of the foot being twisted, it is moved backwards and forwards while you press or thumb walk across the reflex.

● **hooking** Hooking is used to access reflexes which are very deep seated or that are too small in area to benefit from thumb or finger walking. Use the side or top of your thumb to press the point. Don't let your thumb slide off the point and try not to release the pressure – it's a bit like running on the spot. Basically, you are just bending and straightening the first joint of your thumb. Hold the position for a few seconds and then release. This is most effective when working on small reflexes such as the pineal and the pituitary glands, the appendix and the hypothalamus.

full reflexology treatment

● **warm up** You can start by helping to relax the feet and mind of the person you are working on, by what is known as 'greeting' the feet. No, you're not just saying hello, but performing a physical move which establishes contact between the recipient and yourself. Firstly, grasp their feet, thumbs under the sole, fingers resting on the top of the feet, and squeeze them firmly with your thumbs and fingertips. Then repeat by grasping the soles – place your fingers at the base of the toes and the thumbs at the arches. Squeeze for a few moments. The next step is to gently rotate the ankles. Work on one foot then the other. Let the ankle rest in the palm of one hand and use your other hand to manipulate the foot. Roll it one way, then the other. Stretch the foot so that you arch it and flex it alternately.

● **'greeting' the feet**

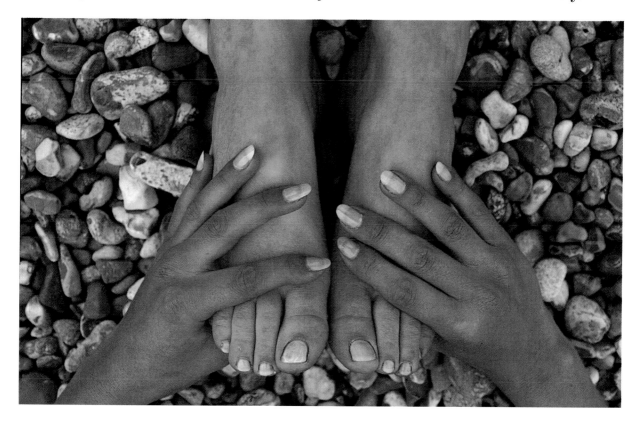

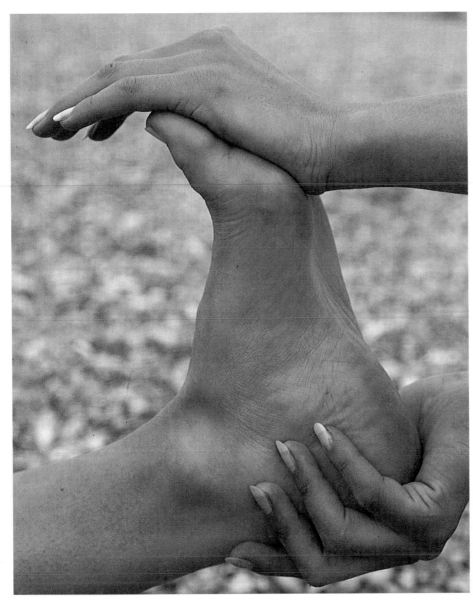

● **rotating the ankles**

the solar plexus reflex on your sole, located about 5cm (2in) below the middle toe. This is one of the main relaxation points. Using your hands, roll the foot from side to side. This boosts circulation and helps to relax the muscles. The heel of the foot should rest on the futon or floor. Finish by using a few soothing strokes across the sole and upper part of the foot. Now you're ready to start the treatment. Start work on the right foot and use thumb pressure to stimulate each point. Use firm but not uncomfortable pressure and hold for about 5 seconds. Then move on the the next point. A full treatment will last about an hour.

Don't push or pull too much – this move should be performed with care. Squeeze one foot so that you press the outer edges together to create a hollow in the sole. Now use a hooking movement and press your thumb into

full foot reflexology treatment

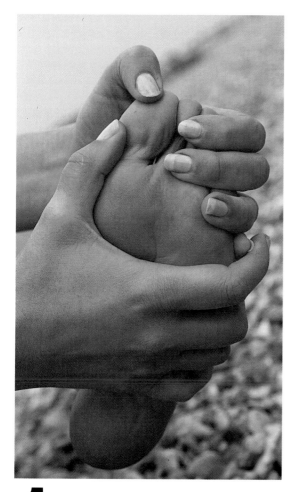

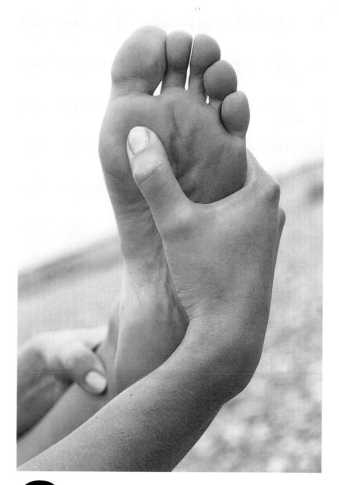

1 Use one hand to gently flex the foot so that the sole is as flat as possible. With your thumb, press across the foot, just under the ball (above) – this corresponds with the diaphragm line on the chart (see page 105). Next, work your way up the spinal zone, starting at the inner heel and moving along the arch of the foot towards the toe.

2 Use both your thumbs to work over the big toe area, massaging the big toe itself, and the soft pad directly in line with it, on the sole of the foot (above). According to the reflexology chart, this area relates to the head, so if the person you are massaging suffers from headaches, it's a good idea to spend a few minutes working on this region. Next, use the same technique on the rest of the toes, working on the top, sides and back of each one.

3 Work now on the upper part of the foot. Use your thumb to press between and along the tendons of the foot, working from the toes towards the ankle (right). This area corresponds to the breasts and chest and by stimulating these points on the feet, you can help to release tension and improve blood circulation in these areas.

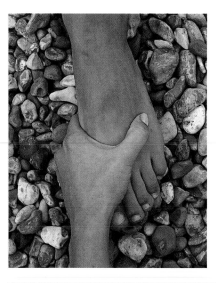

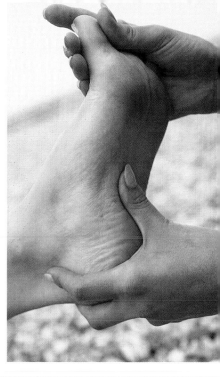

4 Now go back to the sole and concentrate firm thumb pressure over the ball of the foot and under the **big toe** (above far right). This helps to stimulate the lungs. On the left foot, pay special attention to the area just below the ball of the foot, as this relates to the heart.

5 Using diagonal movements, work from the centre of the foot, the waist line, to the upper part where the diaphragm line is located (right). Use the same method to work from the heel to the waist line. This will help to stimulate the workings of the digestive system.

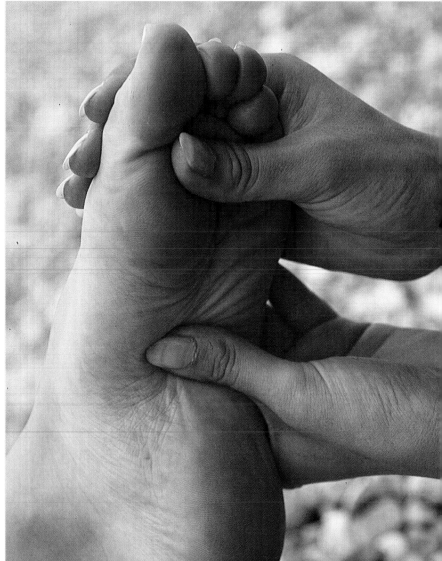

6 **Allow the foot to rest in your right hand while you work around the ankle area with your thumb** (right). **Use your other hand to support the foot while you work. Circle around the ankle bone, first one way then the other. The ankle relates to the lower back, reproductive organs and the legs. Take care when massaging this area, especially if your partner is either pregnant or menstruating. It can be unbearably tender – if it is, it is best to avoid it at these times. (Do not perform reflexology on anyone who is less than 12 weeks pregnant.) Work slowly but surely and regulate the pressure to suit the comfort of your partner.**

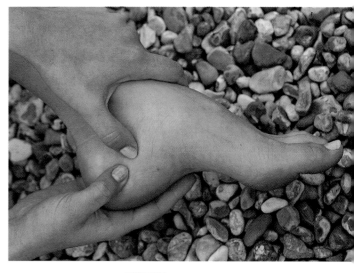

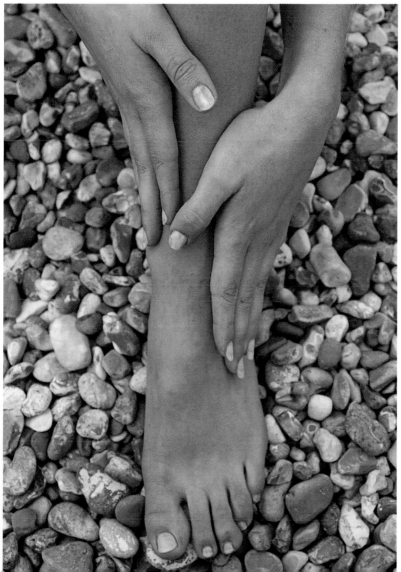

7 **Next, work your way across the whole heel area. If the area is calloused, you'll need to use really firm pressure. Don't be afraid to press deeply, especially if you detect any lumpy areas. Massaging the heel can help to prevent or alleviate lower back pain.**

8 **Finish the reflexology treatment by using the palms of both hands to stroke the foot, working from the ankle to the toes** (left). **Repeat for several minutes. Encourage your partner to rest for at least ten minutes. Cover them with a blanket.**

113

full hand reflexology treatment

Working on the hands is an easy and convenient form of reflexology. As hands are more accessible than feet, they are ideal for performing quick pick-me-up moves. One of the disadvantages, however, is that the reflexes here are deep seated and are therefore much more difficult to stimulate. The hand sequence is very similar to that performed on the foot. The same sort of movements are used although obviously the reflex points are different (see page 106).

Little preparation is needed for hand reflexology. You can run the hands under warm water or rub them briskly between your palms to heat them slightly *(below)*. As with the foot work, you don't need to apply oil or cream but you could apply some at the end of the treatment for comfort and to moisturize .

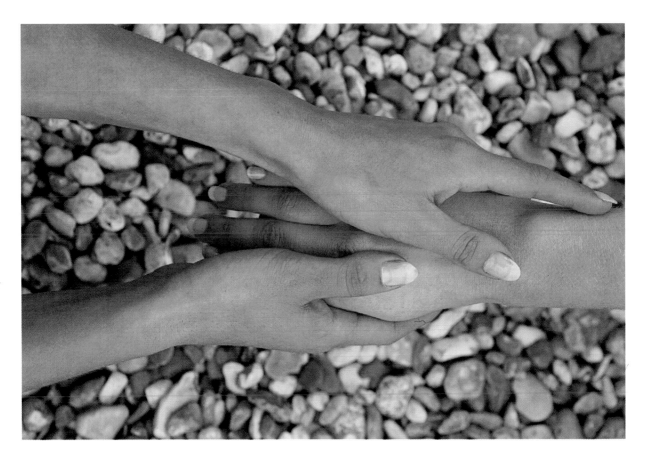

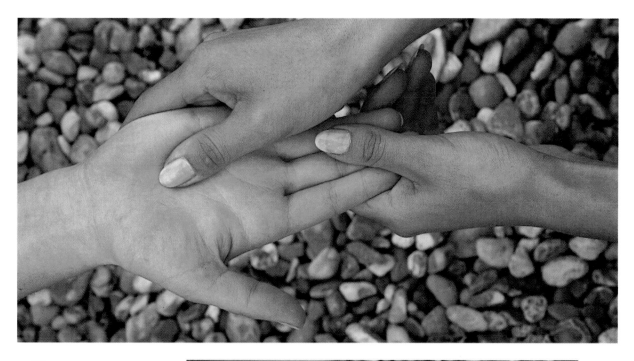

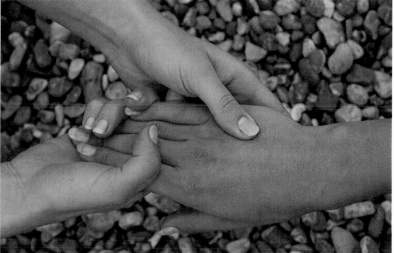

1 Hold the fingers of the hand being treated with one hand and use the thumb of your free hand to press the middle of the palm, where the diaphragm reflex is located (above). Use the thumb walking technique across the line and back. Press the fingers towards the palm of the hand so that you can stimulate the reflex effectively.

2 Now turn the hand over so that the palm faces downwards – you could rest it on a cushion or table (above). Use both your hands to hold the fingers of the hand being massaged. Use your thumb to work down the underside of each finger and between the metacarpal bones on the palm. Repeat on the upper hand.

3 Use your thumb to work across the liver reflex which is located in the middle of the hand, on the soft fleshy part. Work in small steps and use firm pressure. You can also treat this point on the upper hand, but it's not as easy to reach.

4 **Use your thumb to work along the reflex of the lower back to the cervical reflex by thumb walking along the side of the heel of the hand and along the side of the thumb** (right).

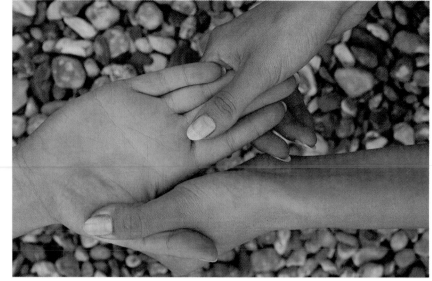

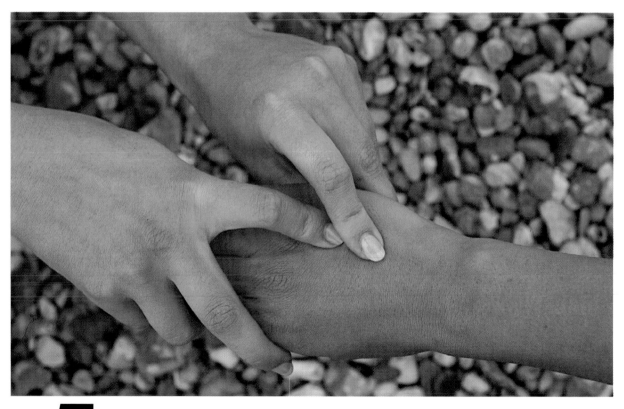

5 **Finally, working on the upper hand, use your index fingers to press along the leg and hip reflex, located at the outer edge of the hand, just below the waist line point** (above). **Use one finger then the other to create an effective rhythmical stroke.**

diy reflexology

Massaging your own hands and feet can be very beneficial to your health – and who knows, you might even enjoy it. You can give yourself a fairly effective treatment, although it may be more difficult for you to break down accumulated crystalline deposits yourself, because the angle of pressure you apply will differ from that given by someone else. Reflexology experts recommend that you massage your feet up to three times each day in order to maintain opti-mum health. While it's a great idea, it's not very practical, so just do it as often as you can.

Position yourself comfortably on a bed, propped up by cushions and pillows, or on a futon on the floor. You can also sit in a chair, if it is more convenient. Rest one foot on the opposite thigh so that the sole is facing upwards. Use the same sequence as before to treat the whole foot area. Then repeat on the other foot. Once you have treated your feet, move on to your hands.

diy reflexology troubleshooters (hands and feet)

Here are just a few useful reflexology workouts, designed to alleviate common complaints. You can use them twice daily on their own or in combination with the full hand and foot reflexology sequences:

colds and flu
Adrenal glands –10 times
Ears – 15 times
Lungs – 10 times

pmt (premenstrual syndrome)
Adrenal glands – 10 times
Brain – 10 times
Kidneys – 10 times
Ovaries – 10 times
Pituitary gland – 10 times
Thyroid gland – 10 times
Uterus – 15 times

stress
Kidneys – 15 times
Lungs – 15 times
Pituitary gland – 15 times
Solar plexus 15 times
Spine – 15 times
Thyroid gland – 15 times
Solar plexus – 10 times
Spine – 10 times

constipation
Adrenal glands – 10 times
Intestines – 15 times
Liver – 15 times
Pancreas – 15 times
Solar plexus – 10 times
Stomach – 15 times

fatigue
Adrenal glands – 10 times
Brain – 10 times
Heart reflex – 10 times (left foot only)
Liver – 10 times
Lung – 10 times

headaches
Brain 10 times
Pancreas – 10 times

insomnia
Brain – 15 times
Solar plexus – 15 times
Spine – 15 times
Thyroid gland – 15 times

menstrual cramps
Solar plexus – 10 times
Spine – 10 times
Thyroid gland – 10 times
Uterus – 10 times

nausea
Brain – 15 times
Ears – 15 times
Intestines – 15 times
Solar plexus – 10 times
Stomach – 15 times
Pituitary gland – 15 times
Sinuses – 15 times

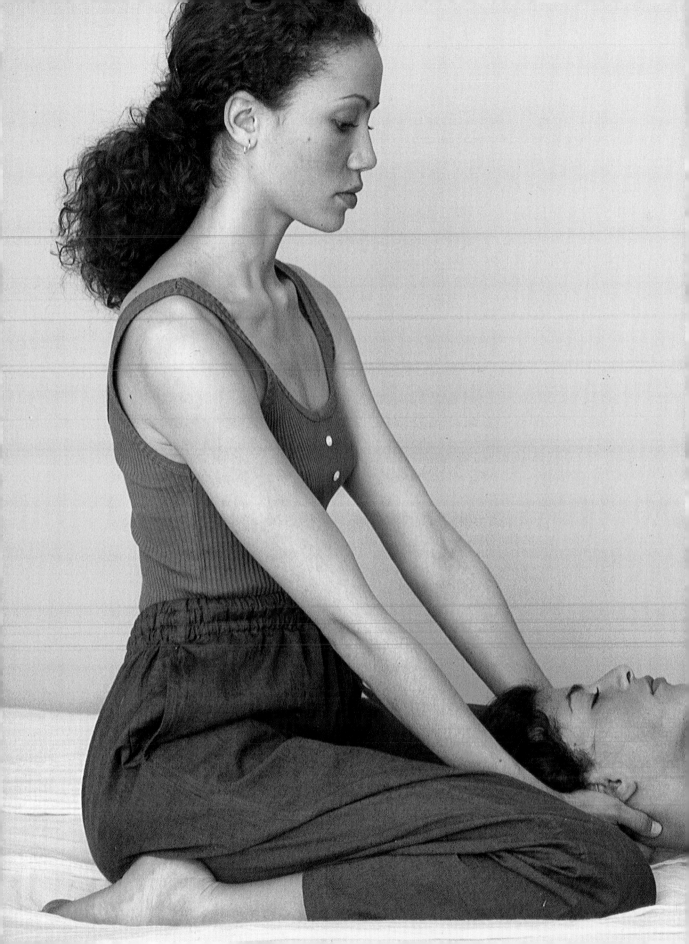

shiatsu

Shiatsu means 'finger pressure' in Japanese and is a combination of massage and acupuncture without the needles.

The elbows, knees and palms of the hands are also used during a Shiatsu massage and stretching exercises, similar to those used in yoga, are performed to improve flexibility and as a warm-up to the massage.

Shiatsu originated in China between 2,000 and 3,000 BC – the Chinese called it *anma*. It was then adopted and refined by the Japanese, who are responsible for modern shiatsu massage. Its main aim is to harmonize and rebalance the body's *Chi* (Chinese) or *Ki* (Japanese), which means energy. Shiatsu practitioners believe that the body has 12 energy channels, or meridians. Pressure is applied to points, known as *tsubos*, along these meridians in order to unblock tension within the body which might cause the *Chi* or *Ki* to become blocked. According to Shiatsu philosophy, blocked energy leads to disease, so regular massage is essential in order to prevent illness.

If you go for a shiatsu massage, the practitioner will look at your body in a holistic way and will watch for areas where there is physical imbalance and therefore a possibility that energy may be blocked. Sometimes this can be seen in body shape or posture and by looking at the face.

shiatsu preparation

Shiatsu differs from most types of massage in that it is practised through a layer of fabric or clothing – so you don't need to undress to have a treatment. Nor do you need to use oils. This makes it a very versatile technique and one that is easy to practise on friends and family. Both the practitioner and the person being massaged should be dressed in light, loose-fitting clothes.

Shiatsu massage is always given on the floor, with the recipient lying on a thin mattress or futon. But you could use a thick towel or blanket instead. The person to be massaged should lie down on their stomach and you should kneel by their side. Allow the massage recipient to get comfortable and encourage them to breathe deeply and evenly.

pre-shiatsu exercise

There are a few basic rules to observe when giving a shiatsu massage. It is very important to use your body correctly as you practise the moves. This will make all the difference to both you and the person being massaged and will help ensure that you don't get tired. It will also mean that the recipient will get the optimum benefit from the session. One of the essentials is to learn how to feel your own centre or *hara (right above)*. To do this, kneel on the floor, with your bottom resting on your heels and your thighs together. Make sure that your back is straight. Fix your gaze in front of you and inhale deeply, taking the air to a point just below your navel. Feel your abdomen swelling as you breath in and flattening as you exhale. Do this for a few minutes.

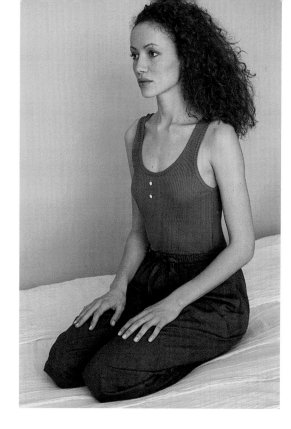

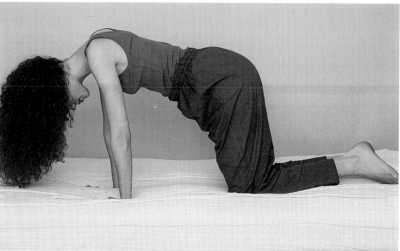

Get down on your hands and knees, legs hip-width apart, hands in line with your shoulders and fingers apart and pointing forward (*above*).

Let your eyes relax and look down at the floor. Don't tense your arms or shoulders – just flop like a rag doll. This effortlessness is what you should experience when you are practising shiatsu.

the tsubos

There are about 600 shiatsu points, or tsubos, over the body, but fortunately it's possible to give an effective treatment using only a fraction of these. The points are named according to the meridian that they lie on, so that their location can be easily described. For example a point lying on the Liver (LV) meridian, will be identified as LV. Then its exact site according to the chart will be given as a number – i.e. LV 3. The point also has a name – Bigger Rushing – derived from its oriental origins. The points can be used in combination to give an overall treatment or as instant troubleshooters. There are also specific points on the face and feet. (See pages 123 and 124).

When you use specific tsubos, treat the points on both sides of the body. Press and hold for between 30 seconds and two minutes and apply pressure in the same way as in the basic sequence. You can either press the point and hold it without moving your thumb or you can use small circular movements, or simply push your thumb in and out. You should press the point as your partner exhales and then gently release the pressure as they inhale again.

We have selected twenty of the most commonly used points which you can press to enhance the effect of the basic sequence or use in combination on their own to troubleshoot specific problems.

1 **Windy Pond – Gall Bladder (GB) 20** – Located just under the back edge of the skull in the hollow between the neck muscles. This point helps to soothe sore eyes, blocked sinuses, alleviate cold and 'flu symptoms, headaches and neck tension. It is also used to treat dizziness.

2 **Shoulder Well – Gall Bladder (GB) 21** – Located on the top of the shoulder in the centre of the large muscle. You'll know you've found it as it may be painful or sensitive. This relieves conditions such as frozen shoulder and can also help during childbirth and to stimulate milk production. DO NOT USE DURING PREGNANCY.

3 **Gate of God – Heart (HT) 7** – Located in the depression on the wrist directly under the wrist bone on the underside of the arm and in line with the centre of the little finger. This point can help to revive an unconscious person, can help cure insomnia, calm hysteria and alleviate high blood pressure and anxiety.

4 **Inside Gate – Heart Governor (HG) 6** – Located three finger widths above the wrist between the tendons in the centre of the underside of the arm. This provides relief or nausea, vomiting, travel sickness and helps cure insomnia.

5 Lung Back Transporting Point – (BL) 13 – Located two finger widths to the sides of the spine and in line with the space between the third and fourth thoracic vertabrae. This point helps coughs, asthma and other respiratory conditions.

6 Kidney Back Transporting Point – (BL) 23 – Located two finger widths to the sides of the spine, in line with the space between the second and third lumbar vertebrae. This point stimulates the kidneys and can also be used to treat lack of sexual desire, physical weakness and exhaustion, depression, chronic back pain, weak legs, ear problems and poor willpower.

7 Large Intestine Back Transporting Point – Bladder (BL) 25 – Located two finger widths to the sides of the spine in line with the space between the fourth and fifth lumbar vertebrae. Helps to stimulate the large intestine and therefore is useful for constipation or diarrhoea, abdominal distension and chronic or acute back pain.

8 Bubbling Spring – Kidney (KD) 1 – Located in the crease in the middle of the ball of the foot. This is a useful point for improving vitality and well-being and for easing feelings of fear and dizziness.

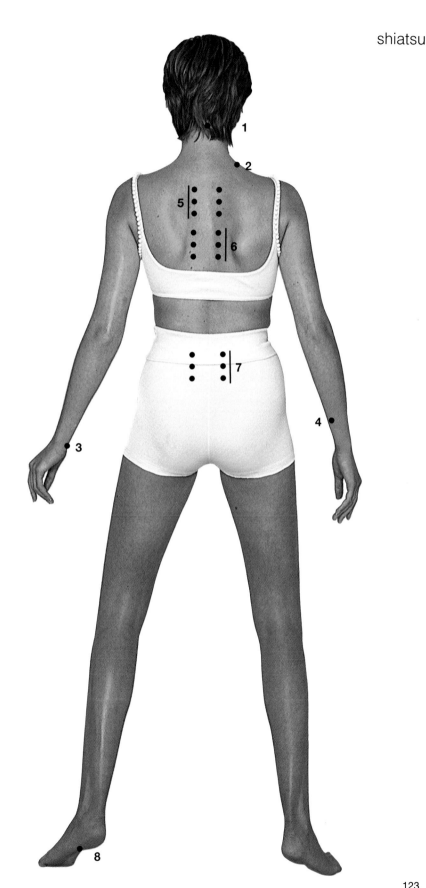

9 Leg Three Miles – Stomach (ST) 36 – Located just below the kneecap in the hollow just above the outside edge of the tibia. This point helps to stimulate the stomach and spleen meridians. It's particularly useful for fatigue, tired legs and loss of appetite. It also helps to boost the immune system.

10 Great Eliminator – Large Intestine (L1)4 – Located on the fleshy part between the thumb and the index finger on the upper part of the hand. This helps to stimulate the digestive system, alleviates constipation and relieves headaches and tension in the hands. THIS POINT MUST NOT BE USED DURING PREGNANCY.

11 Lake of the Energy on the Corner – Large Intestine (L1) 11 – Located at the end of the crease formed by bending the elbow. This helps to relieve hypertension, tennis elbow and haemorrhoids.

12 Meeting Point of the Three Yin Leg Meridians – Spleen (SP) 6 – Located four finger widths above the tip of the ankle bone, just in front of the tibia bone. This helps relieve menstrual pain and reproductive disorders, insomnia, eating disorders and digestive problems. DO NOT USE DURING PREGNANCY.

13 Bigger Rushing – Liver (LV) 3 – Located in the crease two fingers above the first and second toes. This helps ease headaches, dizziness, nausea and muscular tension and improves liver function.

14 Outer Gate – Triple Heater (TH) 5 – Located three finger widths above the wrist in the centre on the top of the arm. This helps to soothe tinnitus, ear infections, migraine headaches and stimulates the pituitary gland.

15 Silk Bamboo Hollow – Triple Heater (TH) 23 – Located at the outer corner of the brow where you can feel a dip in the bone around the eye. This is good for headaches, eye and ear problems.

16 Gate to Original Ki – Conception Vessel (CV)4 – Located four finger widths directly below and in line with the navel. This helps to strengthen our energy levels, improve kidney function, reproductive organ problems and alleviate fatigue.

17 Great Palace – Conception Vessel (CV) 14 – Located a thumb's width below the lower tip of the breast bone – the solar plexus. This stimulates the stomach and heart and helps to calm the stomach. It also has a calming effect on the mind and emotions.

18 Empty Space in Bone – Stomach (ST) 3 – Located in the space under the cheekbone, in line with the centre of the eye. This eases sinus and nasal congestion, facial tension and toothache.

19 Heavenly Pivot – Stomach (ST) 25 – Located three finger widths on either side of the navel. This can help with abdominal discomfort, such as period pains, bowel movements and digestive disorders.

20 Hundred Meetings – Governing Vessel (GV) 20 – Located in the centre of the head in line with the top of the ears. This relieves headaches, dizziness and haemorrhoids.

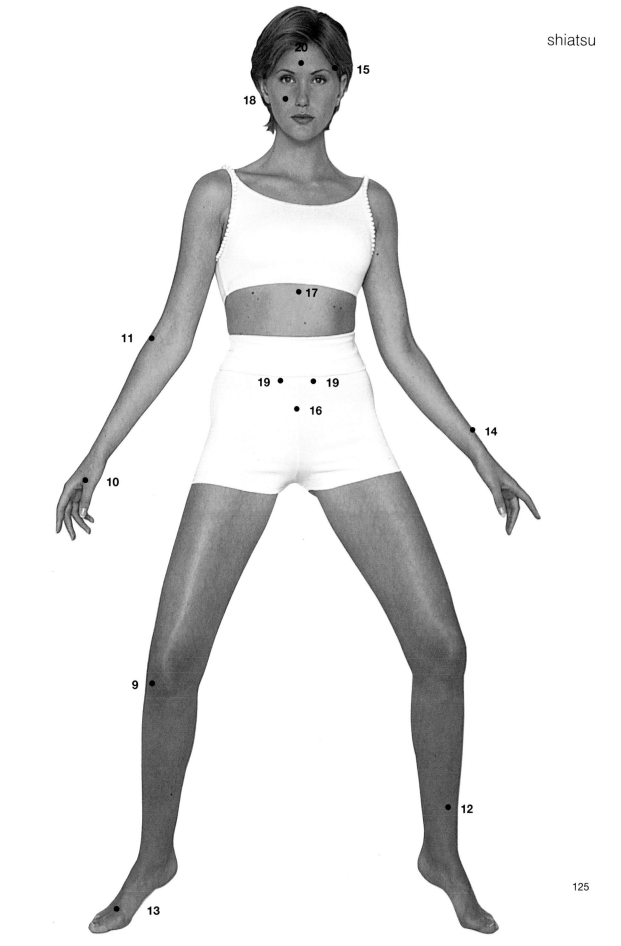

basic movements

Just as in Swedish massage and reflexology, specific moves are used in shiatsu. An experienced shiatsu practitioner uses their whole body during a massage. Elbows, knees, feet and hands are all employed.

shiatsu checklist

1. Make sure that you are relaxed before giving the massage. Do some deep breathing exercises, yoga or meditation before you embark on the massage.
2. Ask your partner how they are feeling before you begin and check whether they have any specific aches and pains.
3. You shouldn't feel any strain when giving a shiatsu treatment. If you do, stop. You're obviously not at ease or relaxed. Take a few minutes to relax before you attempt to start again.
4. As with most types of massage, use your weight and not your strength.
5. As you move from one stroke to another, use your *hara,* or centre, to shift your weight. Don't jerk your body or press down heavily on one side as you move.
6. Always use your weight at right-angles to your partner's body. You need to be on your hands and knees on the floor to do this.
7. Always ask your partner if the pressure is comfortable or if they would like harder or softer pressure.
8. Hold your weight on the body for about fifteen seconds while performing a move or stretch.
9. Make sure that you are using equal weight on both hands.
10. Always move steadily and rhythmically as you go from one position to another. It should feel rather like a choreographed dance.
11. As with other types of massage, always maintain physical contact with your partner during the massage. Don't be tempted to take your hands off the body, even when your partner is turning over.

However, it's not possible in one chapter to describe all the ways in which you can work on the meridians. Start with these basic moves and once you've mastered them, you will have the confidence and skill to learn other techniques. For further reading on shiatsu, see the Bibliography on page 144. As long as you keep the basic principles in mind, such as how to use your weight, you can be fairly creative.

● **thumb walking** Use the ball of your walking thumb to press specific points. Rest your other fingers on the skin to give a firm, steady pressure (*opposite above left*).

● **elbow pressure** You can use your elbow along the back and legs to get a deep, even pressure. Relax your hand and arm to keep the pressure gentle (*opposite above right*).

● **knee pressure** The knees can be used on the thighs and lower legs. Support yourself on all fours, placing your hands on the recipient's body. If you are using your knees on the legs, for example, place one hand in the centre of the buttocks and one hand on the heel of the foot. Then raise one knee and place it on the thigh, spreading your weight across your hands and your knee on the floor. Then use the weight of your body to exert a comfortable pressure.

● **foot pressure**
Using your feet can be a useful way of applying pressure to your partner's feet. When they are lying face down, with their legs about a foot apart, you can slowly and steadily 'step' on to their soles with the balls of your feet (*right*). This is one instance where you can't keep both hands in contact with the body!

● **two thumbs** When you need deep pressure on soft, fleshy areas such as the buttocks, soles of the feet and shoulders, use one thumb on top of the other. Rest your other fingers on the skin to keep a steady pressure.

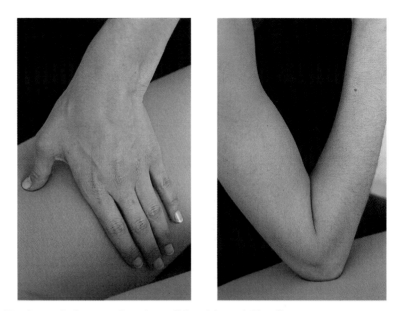

● **Basic techniques: thumb walking** (above left)**, elbow pressure** (above right)**, foot pressure** (below).

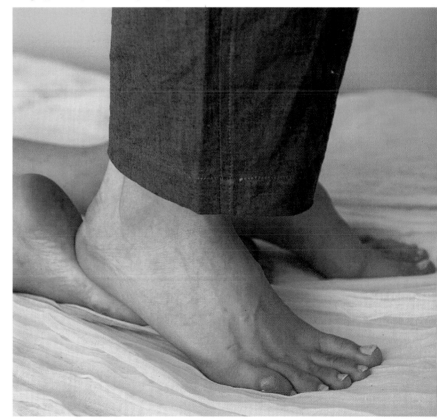

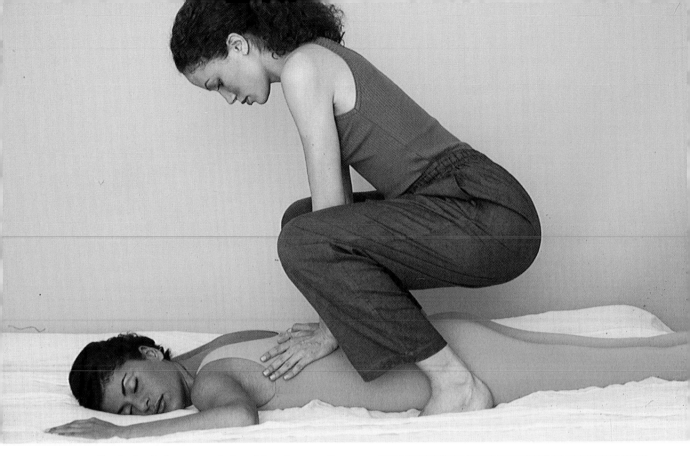

● **Basic techniques: palming** (above)**, pounding** (below)**.**

● **palming** This is one of the simplest, most widely used techniques in shiatsu. With an open hand, you lean your weight on the body *(above)*. Let your hands curve to follow the contours of the body. Use palming before you apply specific thumb or finger pressure to relax your partner.

● **squeezing** When working on the arms and lower legs, you can stimulate the points by squeezing the limbs between your thumb and fingers.

● **pounding** Use your fists to drum on areas such as the hips, the top of the legs, buttocks and back *(right)*.

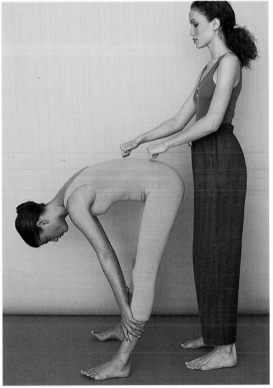

full shiatsu sequence

This is a very basic shiatsu sequence, as some movements have been eliminated for safety reasons. Once you have mastered this sequence, you can go on to include specific pressure points, or *tsubos*, depending on the needs of the person being massaged.

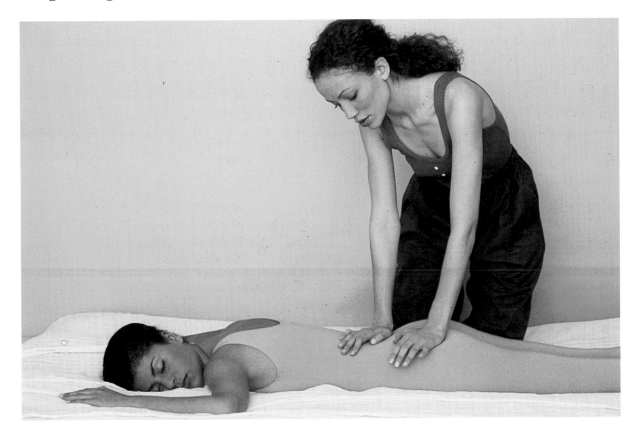

● the back and shoulders

1 Ask your partner to lie face down with their head turned to one side. Kneel by their right side and place your left hand on their lower back (the sacrum). Maintain the contact for a few moments (above). Slowly begin rocking the body from side to side. This helps to relax your partner and allows you to see areas of tension. In most people, the upper back is stiff and requires shorter bursts of pressure and pounding, whereas the lower back is often weaker and will require longer periods of gentle pressure.

2 Move on to all fours, without taking your hand from the back, and place your other hand on the left-hand shoulder. Palm down the back twice and then repeat on the left side.

3 With a flowing movement, step across your partner and place their arms with the palms facing upwards and the elbows slightly bent. Place the palm of your left hand between the shoulder blade and the spine and palm down the whole of their right arm and onto their palm. Repeat this twice. Then move on to the other arm (right).

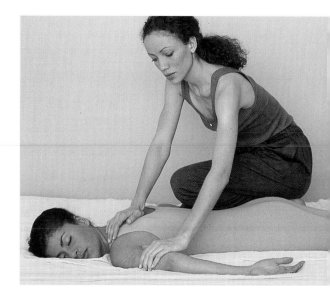

4 Place your thumbs on either side of the spine between the shoulders (right). Lean your weight forwards and hold for between five and fifteen seconds. Move down 3cm (1in) or so and repeat this move. Continue down the back in the same way until you reach the lower back.

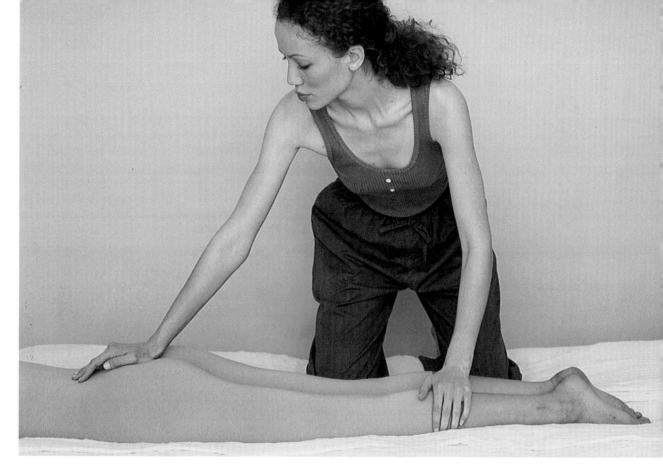

● the bottom

1 Place one hand on the lower back and use the other hand to palm the right hand buttock, working from the top of the buttock and moving down to the top of the leg (above).

2 Keep the hand on the lower back and use the thumb of your other hand to press four points along a line in the centre of the buttock (right).

3 Now repeat both movements (1 and 2) on the other buttock.

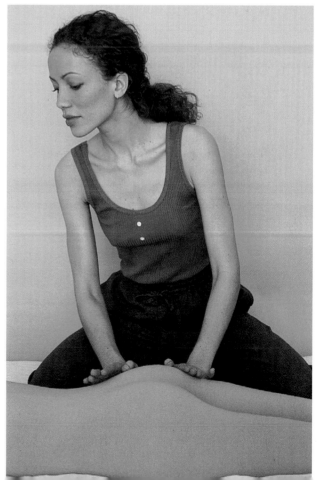

● the legs

1 Step back over your partner so that you are on all fours again. Place your left hand on their lower back and palm down their right leg from the thigh to the ankle. Use firm pressure on the thigh and calf and light pressure on the knee area. If you are having to stretch too far, slide the hand that is on the lower back down to the top of the leg.

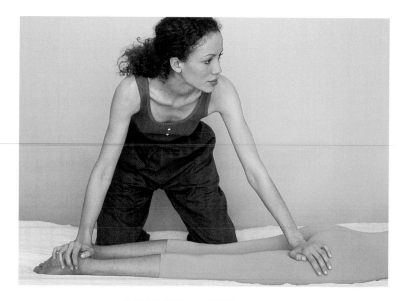

2 Keeping your left hand on the lower back or top of the leg, place your other hand on the right hand heel and press it away from you. This stretches the inner lower leg (above).

3 Repeat the same sequence on the other leg.

4 Now step in between your partner's legs and stand or kneel (right). Hold their ankles and press their feet towards their buttocks for about 15 seconds. Next, cross their ankles and press the feet to the buttocks again. Then repeat, crossing the ankles the opposite way.

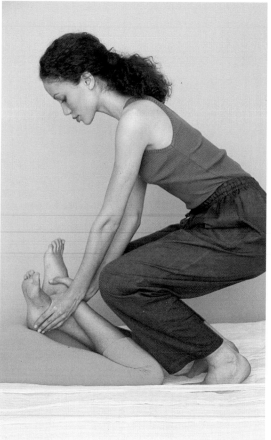

● the feet

1 Keep one hand on your partner and ask them to roll over onto their back. Make sure they do this gently. Kneel at their feet and place one foot on your inner thigh (below). Use the thumb walking technique (see page 126) to press along three of the meridian lines (one on either side of the foot and one down the middle), holding for a few seconds at each point.

2 Hold the foot with both hands and gently stretch the foot by pressing the toes downwards so that they curl under.

3 Next, flex the toes upwards, by holding the foot at the ankle and using your other hand to press the toes up. Reverse the movement so that the toes are pressed down. Repeat two or three times.

4 Holding the foot firmly by the ankle, work on the toes. Work from the little toe to the big toe. Loosely hold the base of each toe between your thumb and your index finger. Use smooth movements to rotate the toe first one way then the other. Then pull it gently away from the foot. Don't worry if you hear a crack! As long as you practise the movements gently, you can't do any harm.

5 Repeat all the movements on the other foot.

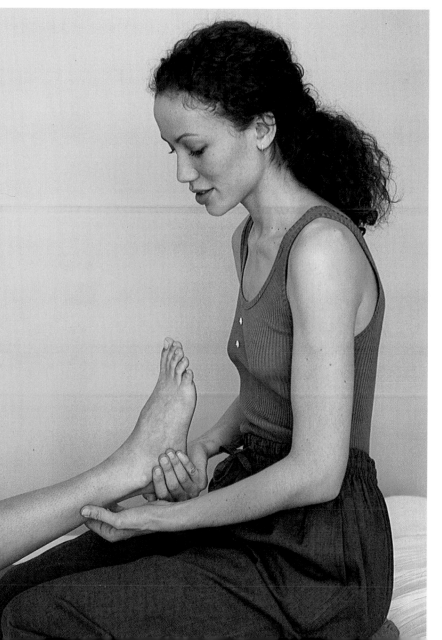

● the legs and hips

1 Move back to your partner's left side, and place one hand on their abdomen. Use the other hand to palm down the front of their right leg, from the top of the thigh to the ankle.

2 Repeat on the other leg.

● the stomach

1 Kneel at right angles to your partner's right side with your knees pressed against their side and leg (below). Put one hand over the other and place them on the abdomen. Use a kneading movement to push gently in to the abdomen with the heels of your hands and then pull towards you with your fingers. Repeat about 15 to 20 times.

2 Kneel sideways with your thigh against that of your partner's and your left arm resting on your leg. Put your left hand under your partner's side, and gently press up. With your other hand, palm around the abdomen starting in the centre, just below and between the rib cage. Move clockwise and press 12 times, as if the abdomen were the face of a clock. Repeat two or three times. Now use your fingers to press a little deeper and follow the same pattern.

3 Finish by pressing just below the navel into the *hara*. Hold for about 15 seconds.

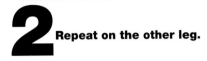

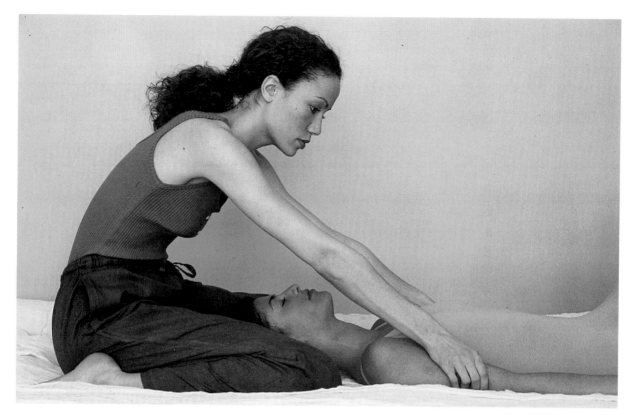

● the chest, arms and hands

1 Move around the body so that you are kneeling on all fours behind your partner's head, with your knees at either side of it. Keep this position for the rest of the treatment. Place their arms out to the side with the palm upwards. Put the heels of your hands to the inside of the shoulder and lean gently forward. Hold for about 10 seconds, rock back and then rock forward and repeat again two or three times (above).

2 Keep one hand on one shoulder and place the other hand on the lower ribs on the opposite side of the body. Lean forwards on both hands to stretch the chest. Move your hand up a few centimetres and repeat until you reach the shoulder. If you're massaging a woman, then move your hand between the breasts for comfort (above right). Now repeat on the other side.

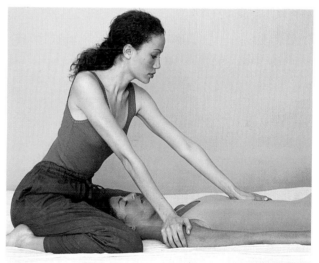

3 Place one hand on the shoulder and use the other down the arm to the wrist. Press lightly at the elbow.

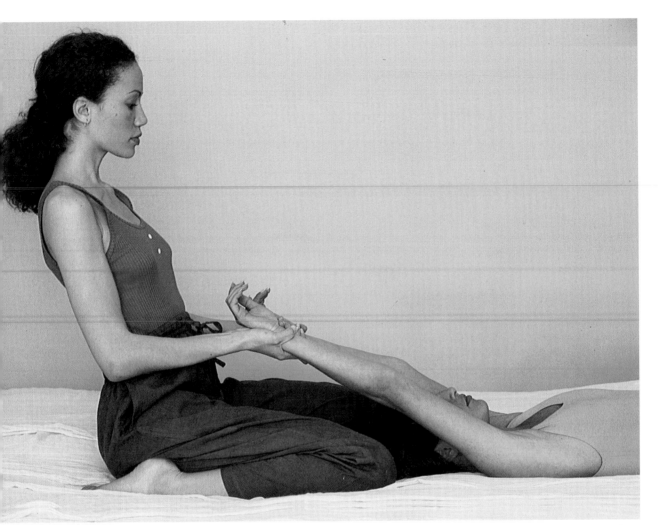

4 Hold the hands by the wrists and lift the arms up. Pull them backwards towards you (above). Lean back to stretch the arms. Hold for a few seconds, relax and then repeat again.

5 Hold the hand with the palm facing upwards and thumb walk down three lines (one on either side and one down the middle). Then hold your partner's hand firmly in one hand and use the thumb and index finger of your other hand to gently rotate and pull the fingers, just as you did with the toes.

6 Place the hand down on the floor and now move to the other side and work your way through the sequence with the other arm and hand.

● the neck

1 Slide your hand under your partner's neck so that the fingers are touching the spine, just below the neck (below). **Slip your other hand under so that both sets of fingers are touching. Gently lift the neck and lean backwards to create a stretch. Hold for 10 seconds, release and then repeat.**

2 Cup your hands and put them on either side of the head with your fingers behind the ears and your thumbs in front. Lift the head slightly off the ground, turn it to one side and gently lay it down,

resting on one of your hands. Using the thumb of your other hand, press into the back of the neck where it meets the skull. Begin behind the ear, move 1cm (½in) or so and press again until you reach the spine.

3 Use your free hand to palm the side of the head. Use your thumb to press four points as you work down — on the bone behind the ear; directly below in line with the jaw; in line with the Adam's apple; and in the hollow where the neck and shoulder meet.

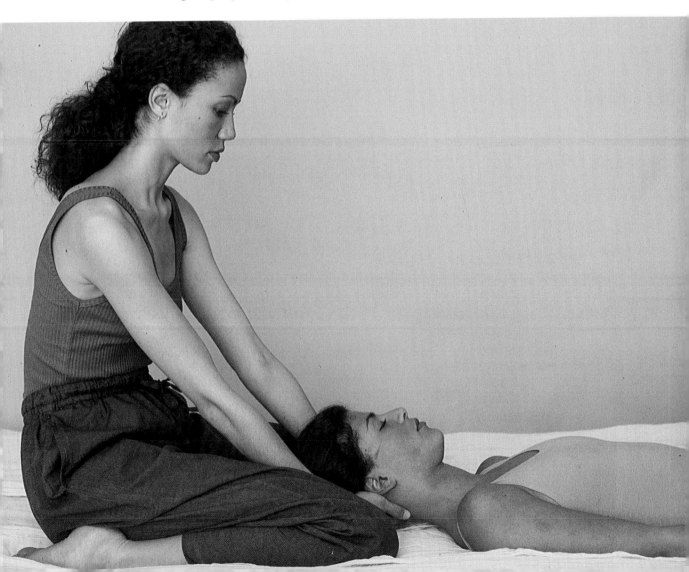

● the head and face

1 Hold the head with one hand. Use the thumb of the other hand to press along a line from between the eyebrows to the crown of the head (below). **Press each point for about 15 seconds, then move your thumb about 2cm (1in) and press again.**

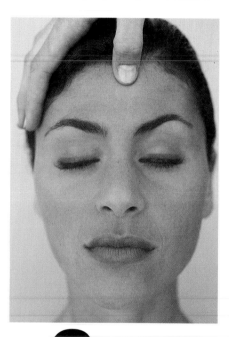

2 Rest your thumbs on the sides of the head and press in two lines as before from the inner edge of the eyebrows to the crown (right). Then follow by working from the inner edge of the eyebrows to the temples.

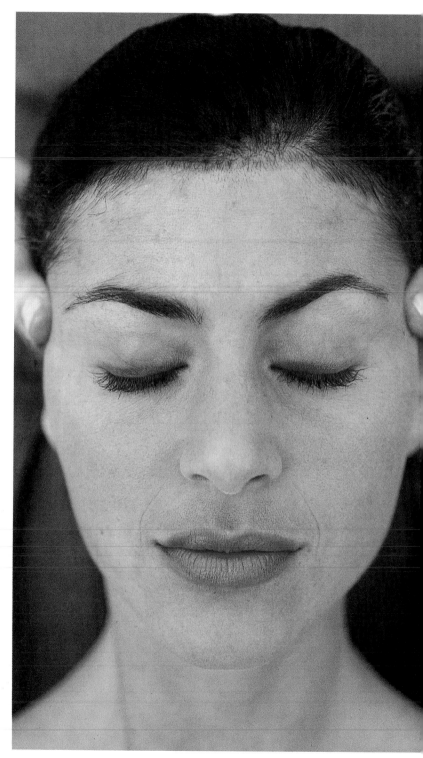

3 Next, work from the inner corners of the eyes along the eyesocket under the eyes and up to the temples. Then follow by placing your thumbs at either side of the nose by the nostrils and work out along the base of the cheekbones.

4 Use one thumb to press in the hollow on the upper lip, just under the nose and then use both thumbs to work out from the upper lip across the upper jaw (right above). **Repeat the same movement under the lower lip, first pressing with one thumb in the dimple between the chin and lip and then two thumbs across the lower jaw and up to the ears.**

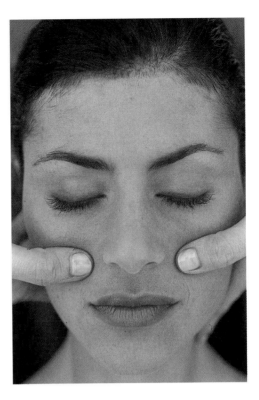

5 Finish the sequence by using the fingers of both hands to press under the jaw, and lean back to gently stretch the jaw towards you (left). Finish by resting your hands on either side of the head by the ears for about 20 seconds and slowly lift your hands away. If your partner wants to lie for a few minutes and relax, cover them with a blanket and leave them until they want to get up.

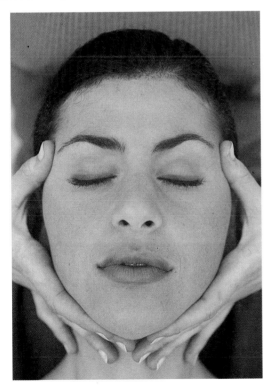

useful addresses

The London College of Massage,
5-6 Newman Passage,
London W1P 3PE

School of Massage,
Freepost,
Manchester M16 8HB

The West London School of Therapeutic
    Massage,
41a St Luke's Road,
London W11 1DD

The Clare Maxwell-Hudson School of
    Massage,
PO Box 457,
London NW2 4BR

International Institute of Reflexology,
PO Box 34
92 Sheering Road,
Harlow, Essex,
CM17 OLT

Reflexology Centre,
18 Deepdene Drive,
Dorking, Surrey

Shiatsu Society,
c/o 14 Oakdene Road,
Redhill, Surrey
RH1 6BT

The Glasgow School of Shiatsu,
19 Langside Park
Kilbarchan,
Renfrewshire
PA10 2EP

The British School of Shiatsu and Oriental
    Medicine,
81 Cornwall Road
Bishopston, Bristol
BS7 8LJ

The Community Health Foundation,
188 Old Street,
London EC1V 9BP

The Churchill Centre,
22 Montagu Street,
London W1H 1TB

index

bibliography

West, Ouida, *The Magic of Massage*, Century Publishing

Harrold, Fiona, *The Massage Manual*, Headline

Brown, Simon and Fletcher, Dan, *Vital Touch*, Community Health Foundation

Worwood, Valerie Ann, *Aromantics*, Bantam Books

Maxwell-Hudson, Clare, *The Complete Book of Massage*, Dorling Kindersley

Brown, Denise, *Aromatherapy*, Headway

Jackson, Adam J, *Massage Therapy*, Optima Books

Norman, Laura, *The Reflexology Handbook*, Piatkus

Cowmeadow, Oliver, *The Art of Shiatsu*, Element

Gach, Michael Reed, *Acupressure*, Piatkus

Lundberg, Paul, *The Book of Shiatsu*, Gaia Books

authors' acknowledgments

A big thanks to Ollie for his hard work and calming presence. Likewise, thanks to Susan at *Cosmopolitan* for all the cups of tea and everything else! Thank you also to Marcelle and Rachel, Vanessa, Anne, Denise, Saskia, Dan, Isabelle and Shirley for their support and contributions; to all the model agents – Greg at Storm, Kelly at Models 1, Sophie at Elite and all the gang at IMG, especially Jonathan – and to all the models for their great patience – Joop, Mark, Nicolette, Jessi, Adir, Carrelyn, Nuala and Khefri; thanks to Suzanna Perks and Karin Darnell for great hair and make-up and to Harold Leighton of Paul Mitchell Luxury Haircare for always being there when we need him! To all at Southern Light Studios, Britannia Row, London N1 and to the Lighthouse Café, Dungeness; thanks also to Madeleine Burbidge and to Stephen Russell and his magic wand.

A final big thank you to all the people and companies who lent us props and clothes – your generosity is much appreciated. For props: The Water Monopoly, 16-18 Lonsdale Road, NW6, tel. 071 624 2631 for the beautiful bath; The Pier, 200 Tottenham Court Road, London W1, tel. 071 637 7001 for chairs; Littlewoods for bedlinen and towels, underwear and bodies; Vivienne Tomei for Jockey underwear; Jackie Cooper for Cacharel underwear; Mary at Fenwick's; Liza Bruce; Top Shop and Next. And not forgetting the following for providing us with massage gadgets, essential oils and carrier oils: Tisserand; the Body Shop; Micheline Arcier and Neal's Yard Remedies.

Pr
an

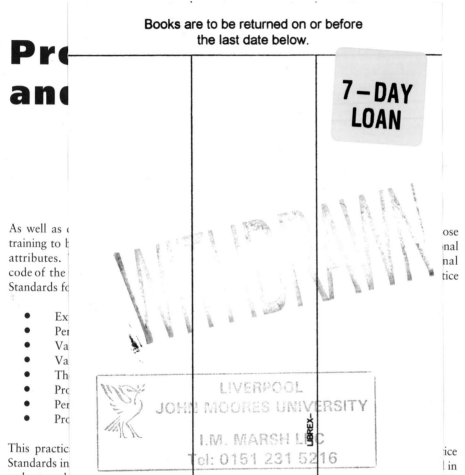

As well as ... ose
training to ... nal
attributes. ... nal
code of the ... tice
Standards fo

- Ex
- Per
- Va
- Va
- Th
- Pro
- Per
- Pro

This practic... ice
Standards in ... in
order to ach.... Practical tasks and questions for discussion are included on each
Standard for use in Professional Studies seminars or during independent study.

James Arthur is Professor of Education and Head of Educational Research at Canterbury
Christ Church University College.

Jon Davison is Dean of Initial and Continuing Professional Development at the Institute
of Education, University of London.

Malcolm Lewis directed the PGCE programme at the University of Bristol from 1996 to 2002,
and is currently PGCE Partnership Co-ordinator and Director of Further Professional Studies.